for Anna,
   departed, but
        never gone.

First published 2023

British Library Cataloguing in Publication Data.

A catalogue record for this book is available from the British Library.

ISBN 978-1-7393100-0-4

Typesetting and origination by Derek Watson.

Cover and Illustration *"for Anna"* by Katherine Donaghy.

Print production by Base Print Solutions Ltd.
Printed by McAllister Litho Glasgow Ltd.
Bound by UK Bookbinders Ltd.

Contents

Introduction

CANCER IS A LONELY PLACE and even though statistically, and frighteningly, 50% of us will be diagnosed with cancer, it is such a desolate feeling when you are told that you have cancer. I was told twice between the start of 2018 and the end of 2019, and each time I felt that it only happened to me.

Like a lot of people, I thought I could handle it with my family, friends and the amazing National Health Service (NHS) teams in Edinburgh and the Scottish Borders. For anyone reading this book who is unaware of the NHS, this is a unique public health service where everyone receives treatment free of charge at the point of delivery, paid for through a National Insurance scheme. In this book you will find many references to the NHS and in part this book is a love letter to the NHS.

It took me quite a while to realise I couldn't handle cancer on my own, as I was missing people who understood what I was going through physically and mentally. As a man I can empathise with my wife, sisters and female friends who describe the pain of childbirth, but I've never experienced it.

I found my cancer family, who are the amazing people gathered by Melanoma UK every Thursday night on Zoom, where people living with Melanoma cancer can share our hopes, fears and funny stories, and this made me realise I wasn't alone.

This book was born from an idea: by asking people to share their cancer stories and what hope means or meant to them, I can help people feel that they are not alone. Whether you are newly diagnosed with cancer, you have been going through treatment, you are living with incurable cancer, or you love someone who has cancer, my hope is that one or some of the stories in this book will help you.

The stories have either been written by the contributors, or I chatted with them over Zoom and a cup of tea, and I then tried to write their story in their own words. Each story gives an insight into how cancer affects our lives, the physical and mental impact it can have, and importantly, it's a timed snapshot of that point in their lives in 2022/2023. I was privileged that people chose to share their stories and in some cases their private feelings that they had not shared with family or friends.

My advice to you in reading this book is not to try and read it all at once. Whilst you may be tempted just to read the stories that relate to the cancer that affects you, or someone you love, by taking your time and reading them all, you may find a bit of hope in a story you might not have considered reading.

Hope is a word which has so many meanings, that are all individual to our circumstances. In collecting these stories, I realise that hope changes shape, colour and texture. For those of us diagnosed with cancer, it can span the first steps of thinking there's something not quite right and we hope it's nothing serious. As we embark on this journey, we might hope it's not cancer, and when it is, we hope that it's curable, treatable, or liveable. For some people with terminal cancer, hope could be that they will have enough time to do things they want, that their end will be pain free or the people they love, and who love them, can manage without them. For those that look for hope, there are also those that lose hope and whilst we can be given hope, it can also be taken away from us.

I knew when I was collecting these stories, that we had to include stories of people that are no longer with us, as sadly this is the reality of cancer, and my greatest hope is if someone was to read this book in fifty–eighty, or one hundred years' time that they might ask *"Did people used to die of cancer?"*

My admiration and respect for everyone who contributed a story can never be measured. People have shared their stories knowing that it might help someone else, and many have shared things that they have never told anyone before. Perhaps I was fortunate that I could relate to some of the physical and mental challenges they had experienced, and they felt that could entrust their story to me.

I also knew that by the time this book was published we could lose some of our contributors, and as this goes to print, we have lost Anna, one of our Thursday night Melanoma clan. The reality is as time goes on more people will depart, but their stories will forever be with us and will keep giving hope. I have tried to include stories of people with as wide a range of cancer as possible, not just Melanoma and where I have interviewed people, I have tried to write their story in their own words.

Hope should be passed on, and with all profits from the sale of this book going to the charity Melanoma UK (Registered Charity Number 1157635), what I ask from you might seem absurd and against the laws of book sales; if this book has helped you, please pass it on to someone else it could help.

Hope is constant.

Kevin

A Model Patient

I **WAS DIAGNOSED WITH KIDNEY CANCER IN JANUARY 2020.** I had been complaining of a pain in the lower right-hand side of my back, which I was putting down to muscle pain due to playing football a few times a week, and sitting at a desk or in the car all day for my job.

My wife eventually convinced me to go to the doctors to have it seen to, which I did in the November of 2019. I was seen by a relatively newly qualified GP. She examined me and said she wanted me to go for a CT scan. I thought I would just be given self-assessed physiotherapy to ease the pain; however, I went for the CT scan in December thinking nothing of it.

Friday the third of January was my first day back at work following the festive break and I was in my car, going for lunch with a colleague, when I got a call from the GP. She advised that they had the results of my CT scan. Everything was clear on my right-hand side, however, they had found a mass on my left kidney. She told me that if I could go home, then I should do so.

At that point my mind was all over the place. I dropped my colleague back at the office and headed home, the whole time thinking the worst and wondering how I was going to tell my wife and kids. My wife works in a GP practice so I knew she would understand from experience what this can lead to, but also understand the process of what would happen next. My daughters were twenty-two and sixteen, my eldest was in her third year of university and the youngest was preparing for her exams. I knew I had to tell them something, but I didn't want to do it until I had more information.

I attended St John's hospital in Livingston in the February for some more CT scans, and I asked the nurse following the scan *"what happens next?"* She advised that I was to go for a biopsy at the Western General hospital in Edinburgh and said something that I will always remember, as it gave me something to pin my hopes to: 'Finding the mass as an incidental find is like winning the lottery as they have caught it very early before it progresses.'

Although this gave me some hope, the wait until I saw a consultant was torturous for my family and I.

I met with my consultant a few weeks later who told me that it was indeed cancer. He confirmed it was a four centimetre mass on the bottom lobe of my left kidney. He reassured me that if I was going to get it then this is exactly what you want as it was slow growing, non-aggressive and on the lobe of the kidney which meant I would only need a partial nephrectomy, and fortunately not a full kidney removal. I remember it as a very confusing day, and it took me some time to take it in. It dawned on me that I might have won a double roll-over lottery, but it was still very early days.

I left that meeting thinking, I could take this diagnosis, as I had imagined a much worse outcome. In a bad situation, I was given good news. It was strange to think of it that way.

My wife and I sat down with our kids and told them what was happening and the fact that they had found it early and it was slow growing. Our youngest daughter was six years younger than our eldest and, as she was doing her exams, we didn't want to distract her but we had to tell her. Knowing they were sisters, they would compare notes.

We tried to avoid negative terms and again focus on the positives, and they were both happy to accept the information we were sharing. They had some questions that we tried to answer. What would happen next? How it would affect me? Would the disease come back? We tried to answer as much as we could, and as honestly as we could.

This is a conversation you never want to have with your kids.

One thing that allowed me to understand it myself and explain it better was a 3D model of my kidney, made for me by the consultant. He had been working on this idea with a colleague and had asked if it would benefit me. I gratefully accepted. This 3D printed model of my kidney and the tumour was really helpful to understand what was happening and in explaining it to my family. Seeing what the tumour looked like, along with the conversations I had with my consultants, meant I could give hope to my family.

I also spoke to my CEO at work, who I had known for thirty years. He had survived an aggressive type of cancer, and he was a great support.

"Don't read too much into what the doctors tell you medically. They won't lie to you and they will try and take the emotion out of your diagnosis as they are very factual, and be prepared or that."

Thanks, Ricky, you added to my hope.

They couldn't do the operation in March 2020, which was when the first UK Covid lockdown happened. My consultant said if they were to operate and I caught Covid while in hospital, there was a good chance I could die, as this disease could attack my major organs. My concern was that a delay could give the disease the time to grow or spread.

I raised my concerns with my consultant about the extended wait, and he advised they would book another CT scan to make sure nothing had changed. During this time, I was put on furlough which gave me more time than I wanted to think about my cancer and imagine what was happening inside. My wife was still working in the GP practice, which during the first wave of Covid, was not a stress-free workplace.

In what seemed like years but was actually a few weeks, I had my scan and results and fortunately there was no change, but in that time between our chat and getting the results, my mind had played many tricks on me.

The surgery was meant to be keyhole, however, due to the consultants not being able to travel to Europe to get training they needed to carry out the procedure due to Covid restrictions, it was advised that it would be an open operation. At this point, I wasn't concerned at how they were going to operate, I just wanted them to remove it. I placed my trust in them.

I got my date for the operation, which was at the same time when we had planned our annual holiday. I was torn between needing the operation and wanting to go on holiday with my family. I tried really hard to convince myself this wouldn't be our last holiday together.

I spoke it over with my surgeon and he said the latest scan was not showing any change and said I should take the holiday, relax, and he would schedule it for November.

This again gave me comfort and taking that holiday made me forget about the cancer when I was there. When I came back I was even more positive and prepared for the surgery and I was incredibly relaxed. I knew what was coming and I now wanted it to happen.

I went in for my operation on Monday 9th November. It was expected to be a two–three hour operation. It lasted nearly seven hours, due to fatty tissue that had formed on the kidney following the biopsy. Apparently, my kidney had responded to the cancer threat by covering itself in a layer of fat to try and protect itself. My body had been trying to fight the cancer.

Waking up in the high dependency unit, I was relieved to hear that they had successfully removed the tumour and they were happy with the results.

I was due to be in the high dependency unit for two days but I was there for a week due to a high temperature. Thanks to Covid, no visitors were allowed and that hit me quite hard. I broke down after five days being isolated from my family.

Once my temperature was under control, the next step was to move into a ward which I didn't want to do as Covid was still present in the hospital. I chose to go home instead. I needed to be with my family at this point and I was allowed to go home.

Nearly two years on from my operation, I still experience pain in my stomach and numbness around the scar area. However, my life has returned to normality with work and family life, and I am back playing football and trying to do what I have always done.

I get checked every year and so far, all is okay. The 'scanxiety' is still there in between the scans and results, and my mind still plays tricks on me.

When positive results come from the scans, the load that's lifted is immense. Consultants remove the emotion from their voice and they sound so calm whilst you're trying to guess what they are about to tell you.

I'm quite a positive person but times like this test how positive you are, not just for yourself but for your family and friends. I needed to be strong at the point of diagnosis and I didn't know if I could be.

As a parent and a husband, I was happy it was me and not my wife or children. I felt I was more able to carry this for them and, yes, cancer has changed my outlook on life one hundred per cent. We have one life and so I'm determined to live it. I don't put anything off until tomorrow.

My story is one of being very fortunate, in catching this early and having strong support around me when it was needed and trying to stay positive. You don't know what's round the corner and if you need to latch onto something, make it hope.

Spread the positivity with your family, be honest, but give them hope.

Andy McGarry

Dad, I'm OK Now

I DON'T VISIT MY GP UNLESS I'M REALLY DESPERATE and I usually 'self-doctor.' How sensible, I hear you not say, when we have a free health service! I usually take it easy for a bit, hope 'things' go away. But some 'things' won't go away. Cancer doesn't, but someone else usually gets that, don't they?

In January, 2020, my wife *made* me book an appointment to see my GP. I had two *suspicious* skin blemishes, only small, on my cheek and neck. No pain, no discomfort or itching, but unlike anything I'd had before. I'd had the mark on my neck for a couple of years. I had it tested once and was told to just monitor it for any changes.

I couldn't see it properly. It was hiding below my ear, like a bloody sniper! Luckily Mrs F could see it and she told me it was changing colour and getting darker apparently. Had I lived alone, I often wonder if anyone would've seen it in time?

Before my GP visit, I did the usual internet research. You will be amazed how many hits a Google search for skin cancer chucks at you. Lots are from sites that have fantastic information and lots with false, incorrect and misleading information. By the time of my GP visit, I had filled my head with fear and anxiety. If you find yourself in this position, please use quality websites like those of the NHS (**www.nhs.uk**) or the British Association of Dermatologists (**www.bad.org.uk**)

My GP is a trained dermatologist. She's quite nice, if a little 'robotic'. She did a visual check, with one of those torch magnifier things. I recall saying, *"It's probably nothing, doc"*. I was shaken by her reply, *"No, it's two skin cancers. We'll have to cut them out"*. She said it so matter of fact, a bit like when someone asks, *"Do you take sugar in coffee"*? She might be an expert on skin issues but I'm guessing she missed the training bit about showing empathy when giving bad news to patients.

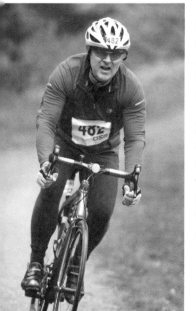

I've had to pass the most awful, tragic news to people in my working life. I was a cop for thirty-one years; major issues can sometimes be our work routines. But I never forgot the importance of being a kind and sensitive human being when passing sad news on. It's the least anyone can try to do! Isn't it?

I left the surgery to tell my wife the news. Driving home that day was really difficult. I went into my appointment feeling quite well and came out of it a cancer patient; and a confused patient at that. I was without any sense of hope or confidence. I told Mrs F the news—heard my voice sounding far more confident than I actually was. My cop training in dealing with trauma probably helped but Mrs F saw through this.

We spent the next few hours talking and helping each other to start coming to terms with my diagnosis.

My kids are grown up, in their thirties and living independently. Telling them wasn't really hard, to be honest. Mrs F and me played things down; I became terribly British in understating it all. We told them separately and emphasised that most skin cancers caught early are successfully treated. They were upset and frightened for me but we all held our emotions in check. The elephant in the room, which was left in the corner, was that a friend of my daughter had died about a year earlier, of skin cancer. We only discussed this sad case much later into my treatment.

I had only one parent alive back then, my dad, Clifford. He was living in a care home, trying to cope with dementia. I'd see a decline in him each time I visited. His speech, movement, concentration and memory were all diminishing. I felt I needed to be the child again and tell my dad. His response was amazing. Telling him my cancer news seemed to temporarily release my 'old' dad from the constraints of his condition. He was very aware of the significance of my news, and asked me several times if it could be successfully treated. When I'd satisfied him it could, he returned back, almost at peace, into his dementia state. For a few minutes someone or something had allowed dad to be able to have the agency to help his son. I found this so comforting and emotional.

About a week after telling dad, his care home went into an early lockdown to try and combat Covid. Remember the government's so called 'protective ring?' Well it didn't help my dad's home. More of this later.

I told a small number of friends at the diagnosis stage, including a public tweet on Twitter. I received a massive number of fantastic tweets from people I didn't know, passing on their experiences of skin cancer and its treatment. Tweeting was a risk but, it let me put the news out in an almost anonymous way first. I was amazed at how common skin cancer is.

The response from my actual mates was a bit of an eye opener. The mates I thought would be forever checking in with me, hardly ever did and those mates I thought would only make an occasional enquiry were messaging me, calling me regularly. I think maybe their personal experiences with cancer probably accounted for this. Or maybe it's my character judging skill!

My next appointment was with a Macmillan nurse, Nicola. After my GP's lack of empathy experience, I expected a similar encounter. It was a complete contrast. Nicola instantly became like a guardian angel to me. She was just the friendliest, easiest person to get on with. Telling her my cancer story and trusting her to help me felt so natural. My GP could learn so much from her. She gave me hope and comfort in spades. I knew I was going to be cared for and receive the best care for my cancers. Mrs F described her as a *"lovely lady"*.

We went through possible causes, with some subtle hinting from Nicola, as there had been from my doctor, that sunbathing could be the cause. I don't sunbathe, never do, it bores me. I've said this so many times to health experts from dermatologists, MacMillan nurses, surgeons, nurses, my GP. I know that none of them believe me. How do I know? Well, being a retired cop I'd spent over thirty years looking in the faces of suspects, witnesses, victims of crime and talking with them. I just know when a person is accepting things as the truth. Apparently cops and car sales people are great at reading body language.

Another possible cause apparently, is trauma. I took a punch once on duty from a guy who found himself 'in the wrong house' (burglar). It connected heavily right on my right cheek, where one of the cancers developed. Who knows, maybe he contributed. What a guy!

I have exposed my face to the sun on a regular basis and I'm a keen road cyclist and walker. I would use sunscreen if it was hot and sunny but hardly ever if it was 'just a nice day'. You know, a sunny warm spring type or autumn sunny day. Now I use sunscreen almost every time I venture outside. Unless it's cloudy or raining, or dark!

The technical bit: My full diagnosis: right cheek (Basal cell carcinoma) and right neck (Lentigo melonoma). Lentigo sounds like an Italian defender who you have to get past to score!

As all of this was happening, a 'mystery' virus was moving around the world in early 2020. Covid was making its presence felt in the UK. I did wonder if this would slow down my treatment at this point, but it didn't. As we all now know the impact of Covid was massive and, as of the time of writing—April 2022, it's still with us.

My operation came swiftly, and a surgeon removed both areas affected. I was surprised at how much physical effort this took him and how vigorous the operation was. He was a really jolly guy and had me in stitches during the op and, of course, afterwards!

A period of treatment, using some powerful cream to clear a tiny trace of cancer cells that still remained, followed for a month. Nurse Nicola warned me the cream would make the area unsightly. It certainly did that! Because of the Covid lockdown my reviews were done by telephone and each time I told Nicola of the mess the cream was causing, she'd say, *"That's fantastic, and exactly what it's designed to do"*.

Now back to my dad in his locked down care home. This is a very sad memory to speak of. I apologise for this, dear reader. As I was nearing my all clear, dad developed Covid and died alone in his home. We were not allowed to go to dad, to hold his hand, tell him we loved him. This will haunt us forever. His funeral was limited to nine of us, for twenty minutes only. No wake or remembrance was allowed.

I never had the chance to tell dad my cancer was now clear. My overriding hope throughout all of this journey, in a perverse way, was that my dad's dementia condition allowed this issue to fade from his conscious thoughts. But I look back at when I did tell him in his home. His almost out of body response was amazing and it struck me how peaceful he was, as he returned to his dementia condition satisfied I was being cared for.

I check myself regularly for any skin or body changes and encourage my family and friends to do this. I use sunscreen daily, as do my family. I said at the start of this story I was a reluctant visitor to my GP, well not any more. If I have any cause for concern I won't hesitate to seek medical advice early!

Mark Clifford Fitzpatrick

Looking Between the Cracks

IT'S NOT ALWAYS EASY TO FIND HOPE WHEN YOU'VE GOT CANCER. We know it's a thing you're meant to do—people say: 'there's always hope'. It's like when they say 'stay positive'—it can be easier said than done. Then we feel bad if we're having a hopeless or negative day. But that's okay. Hope sometimes falls through the cracks. But it's still there.

Thinking about my own cancer journey, it feels like three distinct stories going on at once: the physical, the mental and the emotional. All have had their challenges, and it feels like we need to cope with all of them to get through.

On the physical side, my cancer probably began a few years before I was diagnosed, which was in April 2019. I'd had at least two or three years where I'd felt bloated, very windy, lots of discomfort and lacking energy. Looking back at my GP record, I raised concerns about this 'change in bowel habits' on at least three occasions, and it is a regret that I wasn't referred to a specialist during that time. I've been told since that I 'didn't meet the criteria' to be seen as a cancer risk—but clearly, the cancer was growing inside me, so the criteria were wrong.

In December 2018 I had what I thought was food poisoning, leading to vomiting and then diarrhoea for several weeks. I was finally referred to a specialist in January 2019—who bluntly told me that he didn't think I should have been sent to him. I had a scan, then waited several weeks for a flexible sigmoidoscopy (a kind of colonoscopy, where a camera is inserted to look at your bowel). After this, I was told there was a 10cm tumour in my large bowel, and that I was stage three. An operation was planned for a month's time, but after a couple of weeks I started throwing up and suffering abdominal pain. I was taken to hospital and told I had a blocked bowel—'life threatening'—and had an emergency operation the next day. Most of my large bowel was removed, though the surgeon skilfully managed to connect me up, so I don't have a stoma.

During a three week stay in hospital, I was told that I was now stage four. I wept in the arms of a nurse. I started six cycles of chemotherapy in July 2019. For me the blood test known as CEA has been a good marker of the level of my cancer. Prior to the operation, it was one hundred and twenty, afterwards it was ten. The average is three, hence there was still cancer in me which is why chemotherapy was started. By December 2019 it was down to three.

For the next couple of years, I was seemingly 'no evidence of disease', but the CEA climbed slowly at every quarterly blood test. In February 2022, a scan finally showed what we suspected, that the cancer was back. It returned in my peritoneum (abdominal cavity), an area where chemotherapy hasn't had great success. A procedure called HIPEC—in which the abdomen is opened, cancer cells cut out then heated chemo sprayed inside—is the go-to treatment at this point, as it offers hope and can even be curative. But guttingly, I was turned down as it was deemed to be too risky, with the cancer near to key organs and a major blood vessel.

This was a massive blow.

Losing HIPEC took away any real chance that I'd be cured, and it also meant that any chemotherapy treatment now would be palliative—ongoing—and simply trying to keep me alive. As someone who has always been positive and optimistic about my chances of survival, this hit hard.

Which brings us to the mental challenges of dealing with cancer, of which there are many. When I first found out I had a large tumour, it was obviously devastating. My immediate response, being a glass-half-full person, was 'what can we do about it?' I, with a lot of help from my wonderful wife Julie, threw myself into finding answers. I read books about cancer survivors, and research papers—that I usually couldn't understand—about the causes and treatments for cancer. One of the best things we did was join a Facebook group for stage four bowel cancer. The support and information you can get on there is invaluable.

I tried everything. More exercise, a better diet, Chinese herbal medicine, acupuncture, strange and unknown supplements, meditation, yoga, qi gong, pilates, shiatsu, reiki, reflexology. My brain was saying 'do something', while at the same time, the statistics—for stage four bowel cancer—are saying 'nine out of ten of you will be dead within five years'. I felt I had to be—and would be—the one in ten. But how? Would any of these things make a difference? Was there proof they would work? Even if there wasn't, were they worth trying anyway? Then I found that I couldn't stick with most of them, and felt bad about that.

I was also dealing at first with a lot of anger. We were angry that the GPs had 'missed' my cancer—had even one of them in those previous three years referred me to a specialist, the cancer would have been caught much earlier. Also anger at how slow the process was after I was referred—they clearly knew from my CT scan that I had a large tumour, but it took many weeks before the flexible sigmoidoscopy. It turns out that the delay was because an order of drugs they needed hadn't come through. Because of that, I went from stage three to stage four—basically it seemed like I've been given a death sentence because someone hadn't ordered a damn drug. But there were other delays too—even when diagnosed, there was to be a month before the operation—which when the cancer was clearly progressing so fast, seemed way too slow. And so it turned out, as the blocked bowel nearly killed me.

One key lesson from all of this. If you're like me, you never want to make a fuss, never want to bother people. Often through no-one's fault, things don't happen until you chase them. Make yourself a (polite) pain in the arse—don't let them forget you.

As well as anger, there's also a feeling of guilt. What did I do wrong which means I got cancer? I never smoked, but perhaps I've drunk too much. I've had a lot of red and processed meat in my time, was that it? Too much sugar? Or was it stress caused by a difficult family life? The questions are endless but unanswerable; ultimately just self-torture.

Which feeds into the emotional burden of all this. For me, finding out I had cancer pushed me into strange areas. While in hospital, I started obsessing about reincarnation—if only it existed, that would be okay. But what if I came back to a life worse than this one? I tied myself in knots for a while.

I'll be honest—in the previous few years, because of a difficult home life parenting a disabled child, and perhaps influenced by the cancer growing inside me, I'd battled with stress, depression and suicidal thoughts, but in hospital, knowing the cancer was trying to kill me, those suicidal thoughts disappeared. I didn't want to die.

I think my main emotion though was sadness. Perhaps we don't always think too much about what we've got, or what we could lose. At that time though, my feelings became very clear—leaving behind my wife and our son was too much to bear. The sadness I felt thinking about it was devastating. And motivating—I'd do anything to prevent it from happening.

For me, then, I think I went into 'I'm going to beat this' mode, which came across as a very positive attitude. Even knowing the statistics, even having been told 'you've probably got one to three years', I think I ignored all that.

As mentioned before, having a 'positive attitude' is something that comes up a lot on a cancer journey. I think people want you to be positive—'need' you to be positive. We're told all the time: 'you've got to fight this', 'you can beat this', 'you've got this'. Which in one way is motivating. Perhaps it's like a soldier being sent off to war by cheering crowds—once the cheers fade and you're on the battlefield, all you're trying to do is stay alive. 'You've got this?' No, I really haven't. I'm just doing my best.

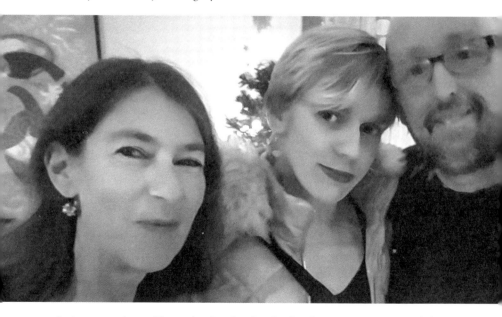

An important lesson I learned is that there's a thin line between 'positivity' and 'denial'. For the first few months, I was being positive—but probably also denying the reality of what was happening. My wife, as usual, brought 'the real'—it wasn't fair on her if I blindly carried on thinking everything will be fine. We needed to prepare for what, statistically, was most likely to happen. And while that may sound negative, it isn't—it meant that we started thinking about all the good stuff we could get on with doing. So yes, we updated my will and made sure bills, etc. were in her name, but we also went to Costa Rica on holiday and blew the savings on a campervan.

Since the cancer returned earlier this year, all those emotions surged back. Fear—first glance at the statistics said the average lifespan for peritoneal cancer is six months. Anger—why didn't they pick up that it had returned sooner? Sadness—despite being 'real' about my prospects, I somehow still believed that I'd be that 'one in ten'. But now, probably not.

I've regrouped again though, and re-found my hope. I'm on palliative chemo, so who knows what will happen. I've always thought that the longer I can stay alive, the more chance there is that a new treatment will emerge that can save me. I still believe that it will. Meanwhile, I'm still completely motivated to stay around for my wife and son.

Hope is not just for the future, it's for the day-to-day moments. Laughing with my wife gives me hope. A tender moment with my often grumpy teenage son gives me hope. Rekindled friendships with people I haven't seen for a long time gives me hope. Pottering around the garden and looking at the life in the pond I built gives me hope. The belief that West Ham will one day win something gives me hope!

I also hope that my story somehow helps others. I talked to the GP and the hospital about the mistakes that were made, and I believe that they will try to ensure they won't happen again. I hope that after hearing my story more people go and get themselves checked out. I hope that medical science finds a way to increase early detection of bowel cancer.

We're surrounded by hope, even if sometimes we have to look between the cracks.

Chris Pitt

Running Into Cancer

I **N THE EARLY MONTHS OF 2017** I was training to take on one of the world's toughest ultramarathons: Comrades, in South Africa. I'd completed the race the previous year and wanted to have another crack at it as you get a special medal if you complete two on the trot. Comrades is 56 miles long, 6,500 feet of climbing and it's usually 28-33°C. It's brutal!

In the February that year I hit the grand old age of sixty but I also hit the start of what would end up being news that would shatter my world. I was competing in the Anglesey half-marathon when, on a downhill section near the start, I felt a searing pain in my right groin. Once onto the flat though the pain subsided. However, over the following weeks, it gradually worsened and I was managing the pain with painkillers because runners are idiots and we always believe we can run the pain off.

At the start of April I completed the Manchester and Paris marathons, a week apart, as training runs for Comrades but the pain in the aftermath was horrendous and I realised that I wouldn't be running Comrades on June fourth unless I did something about it. I made an appointment for May eighth to see a sports injuries doctor and a MRI scan was arranged.

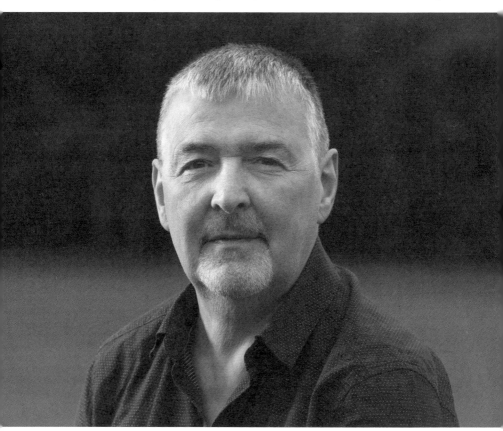

The doctor and radiographer were in and out of each other's offices for an hour or so and it was pretty obvious that they were talking about me, mainly because I was the only person there! When the doctor called me into his office he said, *"We're not seeing what we expected on the scans and want to rule out anything untoward so I'd like you to have blood tests and a chest x-ray straight away. Tomorrow I've booked you in for a full-body CT scan."* As you'll have gathered, I had private medical insurance. Even the NHS at its best doesn't do this that quickly!

As you can imagine, this was terrifying. Even an idiot like me didn't need Mr Google to tell me that you didn't need these for a groin strain.

I went to running club after the CT scan and tried to play it cool but the nerves were absolutely shredded. After our run we were just leaving to head for the pub and a quick beer— well we have been described as a drinking club with a running problem—when my phone rang. I didn't recognise the number so I rejected the call. Thankfully the doctor was persistent and rang again to break the news to me that he was ninety-nine per cent certain that I had prostate cancer and was calling to tell me because he needed me to have further urgent diagnostic tests as soon as possible.

I must have looked ashen faced as a club mate asked me what was the matter and I told her before running to my car and driving home in floods of tears to break the news to my wife.

Ten days of scans, biopsies and appointments with urologists felt like a blur before I was told that I had advanced stage prostate cancer, it wasn't curable, and I might only live two years.

Our world fell apart. All I could think about was dying. Would I get to see my three-year-old grandson, who I dote on, become a teenager? Would I get to walk my daughter down the aisle? And strangely, would I still be able to run?

Here I am five years on and still stable. I've responded superbly to a new treatment that was announced at a conference in 2017 and my insurers agreed to fund for me. I may get to see my grandson become a teenager. I've had two more grandchildren as well. I've walked my daughter down the aisle and yes, I'm still running. I dared to hope that I might get to do those things and a lot of my hopes have been fulfilled. I'm a lucky man I know but I'm making sure I use that luck to lead the best life.

Since starting treatment, lots of new drugs have been developed. I live in hope that, when my current drug stops working—which it will—one of these new drugs will keep me alive and then I hope that more new drugs will come along and, who knows, maybe even a cure. The longer I'm stable the better my chances and I'm firmly of the belief that, without hope we are hopeless.

Tony Collier BEM

Joan, my Ark

I HAD CONVINCED MYSELF THAT I WOULD DIE. It just seemed logical. It was 2006 and at the age of forty-four my experience of cancer, or the Big C as my parents and grandparents called it when I was growing up, was that once diagnosed all thoughts turned to life without my great aunt, my uncle or grandmother. People just died in the nineteen sixties, seventies and eighties once they were diagnosed.

Cancer was a killer and I now had it.

The wee lump on my neck had started to grow and like most men, I had put off any thought of going to the doctor with it. It will go away or just take care of itself.

"Get your f'in arse to the doctors now, Ricky." My wife's friend, who is a brilliant nurse, had seen the lump on my neck six weeks previously and now noted how much it had grown.

She was right and I had put it off, hoping it would go away, but even more, by ignoring it they couldn't tell me it was cancer, could they?

Cancer happens to other people, but surely it won't happen to me?

Well it did.

The oncologist told me the diagnosis and even though I was gobsmacked, my health had taken a recent dive and it made sense.

Squamos cell carcinoma. It's not easy to say and even harder to treat. The cancer was in my throat and was making it harder to eat, drink and talk.

We had no idea if it had spread and if I was to live—they needed to treat the cancer and operate, but they didn't know which to do first.

I was sat in that clinical room whilst the experts discussed what to do first. I must have blended into the furniture, as it felt like I wasn't there. They were discussing my chances of life or death, the various procedures and likelihood of survival, yet I had no part to play or decisions to make.

I needed to know.

My wife Joan sat by my side and I needed to know, *"Will I die from this cancer?"*

The oncologist looked at us and said there were various stages I had to go through and they would evaluate my progress.

Now I'm a black and white sort of guy, and this answer wasn't what I needed to hear.

"In your opinion, and given your experience of patients in similar circumstances, will I die?"

The best answer I got was that without the treatment and surgery I would likely be dead in the next six months.

I don't think oncologists like to paint a pretty picture and it's not their job to present you with a basket of hope, but I appreciated his honesty.

So it began.

The Edinburgh Cancer Centre became my new office, Monday to Friday for seven weeks I went there for radiotherapy and chemotherapy.

People tell you how amazing cancer nurses are and it's hard to put into words how they made Joan and I feel. We were the focus of their day and they took amazing care of us.

I wasn't the only one receiving treatment for this type of cancer and I soon got to know the other patients in for their treatment. We talked about our cancers, the treatment, football, our families and lots of other subjects. You create a bond with those that are going through similar treatment, since they know what it feels like. The hope and fears are shared.

My hope began to fade over those weeks. Like my favourite Hibs top which I'd had for years, the colour begins to go, it starts to fray and eventually it's completely done. My hope started to disappear.

One day the nurses suggested I go to the Marie Curie centre for some respite, but to me this was the last stop for cancer patients, and I thought if I went in I wouldn't come out. It sounds irrational but that's cancer, it plays tricks on your mind.

Soon my friends in the cancer centre started to disappear.

"Where's John today?"

"I'm afraid the treatment didn't work for him, he won't be coming back."

"Not seen Sarah for a while."

"Sorry, Ricky, she died last week."

Everyone I had got to know had died or were dying.

I did not get to know anybody who had successfully beaten this cancer, so why would I be any different?

For those of us with cancer, there can be no harder conversation than the one you have with your kids. Aged ten and sixteen, what the hell was I going to tell them?

I was conscious that my ten year old daughter's best friend had lost her dad to cancer the previous year, and another kid in her class had lost their mother. It had such an impact on the class that the school had brought in bereavement counsellors to help.

I had to tell them there was a chance I wouldn't be around soon. A conversation I hope you never have to have.

I prepared myself to die.

Not Joan.

"You are NOT going to die."

Every day she told me that, as the cancer treatment did its best and its worst and I grew weaker and thinner. I was having to be fed through a tube in my stomach.

Joan was convinced we would win. She set a reminder every hour to make sure I fed myself, and kept fighting.

"You are NOT going to DIE."

It wasn't a wish or a request, she was ordering me not to die.

She built my confidence day by day and I clung on to her hope. The staff would tell me how well I was responding to the treatment, but it didn't sink in that I might win this battle.

Joan knew though. I know there were days when she would be in the room next door, crying and fighting for both of us, and there was no way she was going to let the cancer win.

Day by day, week by week, the treatment did what the oncologist had hoped it would and eventually I was well enough for the surgery.

A neck dissection was needed to remove the lymph nodes to check if the cancer had spread. It was an easy decision for us to go ahead, even though it would permanently change my appearance. The surgeon explained that more men than women went ahead with this procedure, which was difficult for me to understand at the time, but it makes sense now.

They took a large section of my neck and confirmed that the cancer was present in two of the lymph nodes and if these hadn't been removed, it would likely have spread.

The monthly checks soon turned into three monthly then six monthly over the next five years and I still remember the anxiety of waiting on the results, and having Joan by my side, assuring me it would all be okay.

This all started fourteen years ago, and although my cancer has never retuned, there is always a concern that one day, it will.

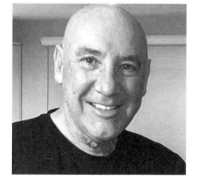

How did I cope with this, I often ask myself?

The answer is easy.

Joan, my Joan, my ark.

Ricky Nicol

Hope, It's a Family Thing

IT IS 29 OCTOBER 2021. I am sitting in a small cubicle in my local hospital. A concerned A&E doctor is gently speaking to me, his face contorted with awkwardness, his voice shaky. *"Stage four metastatic melanoma"*, *"inoperable"*, *"multiple lesions and tumors"*, *"I'm so sorry…"*

My first brush with melanoma came almost twenty years ago when I discovered a strange, black lesion on the left side of my back. I hadn't really noticed it before, since it was situated almost under my arm, and I couldn't be sure how long it had been there. After a couple of weeks of intermittently wondering what to do about it I eventually dragged myself down to the doctor's surgery. He wasn't particularly worried, despite the lesion's strange appearance, but agreed to remove it, whilst taking a biopsy that would be sent for routine analysis.

Months later, when I had almost forgotten about the incident, a frantic call from the GP confirmed that I needed to come into the surgery straight away. I was met by the head of the practice who confirmed that it was a melanoma and required immediate treatment. I felt terrified as all the hopes for my future life fell apart; knowing little about the disease I imagined the worst. I was a wife, mother and teacher; people needed me, relied upon me; this surely could not be happening.

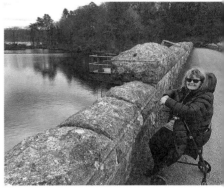

Within two weeks, I found myself in a ward at Saint Bart's Hospital in London having a wide excision on my back and investigative procedures into the related lymph nodes. I was quickly informed that the melanoma was shallow, had not spread, and there was no nodal activity. My relief was indescribable. Hope sprang anew as I realised that I could return to normal life except that I would now need to take far more care when exposed to sunshine, especially in terms of sunscreen application and wearing appropriate clothing. I returned to Saint Bart's for the next five years, receiving a clean bill of health on every occasion. I still went on holidays to warm places but was incredibly careful regarding sitting in the shade, staying out of the midday sun, wearing suitable attire and always using factor fifty sunscreen.

Just as the hospital gave me the all clear it so happened that I moved out of London to Swindon. When I joined a new GP practice I was asked to complete a detailed form concerning issues about my health but also those of my close relatives. When my new doctor read the information, he felt concerned about the amount of cancers that had occurred in relatively young people in my family, including that of my late sister. Consequently he decided to refer me to a geneticist at the Churchill Hospital in Oxford.

My first visit to the geneticist was somewhat disconcerting; I was asked some very strange questions, for example, *"Do you find it difficult to find hats that fit you?"*. It turned out that my head was somewhat on the large side for a woman, and this was possibly indicative of a certain disease, especially when put together with other medical factors including the family cancers. It was suggested that I may have a genetic disease called 'Cowden's Syndrome' and this predisposed me to developing certain cancers across my lifetime, including melanoma. As a consequence, I was to be given yearly scans on various parts of my body (thyroid, breasts, womb, ovaries, kidneys) in order to check that no disease was present, whilst my skin would be thoroughly checked for cancers too.

Over the next ten years I regularly attended appointments and no further problems were found, either in my organs or skin. However, a groundbreaking discovery in the burgeoning field of genetics was made during this period, with one aspect being particularly relevant to me. A genetic variant, called MITF, had recently been linked to the likelihood of developing melanoma. When the Churchill asked me if my blood could be tested and analysed for the presence of this mutation I automatically agreed, and it was quickly discovered to be present. Despite this I remained hopeful about the quality of my life; I was regularly cared for by the hospital as my condition was being constantly and consistently monitored. Even with the arrival of the pandemic, the hospital kept up my routine appointments and I felt lucky to be looked after in this way.

In the summer of 2021, a problem in my back, which I believed to be arthritis, became gradually worse and I presumed that I had a deteriorating spinal issue of some sort. In increasing pain and fearing that there was little hope of getting an NHS appointment any time soon, I was forced to opt for a private back consultation in late October. The doctor assured me that I had all the signs of disc degeneration; he did not suggest a scan, just the usual regime of medication and exercises to follow. On the very same day I had a blinding headache, an unusual occurrence, which left me slightly confused and also feeling that I had undergone a change in my personality. I couldn't laugh or smile and felt that something apocalyptic was taking place.

The next morning, feeling very concerned, I obtained an emergency appointment with my doctor. Worried about my symptoms, he immediately sent me to A&E and I spent several hours waiting my turn to be seen. I was then given both a head and body scan and very swiftly the worst was conveyed to me. Alone, with no relative for support due to hospital pandemic rules at that time, I was told that I had experienced several bleeds on my brain and there were various lesions in it and tumours across my body—notably not in the organs that I regularly had scanned—that were most likely inoperable. At that moment I felt numb, uncomprehending and defeated. The doctor appeared to be signing my death warrant as he admitted me to the ward, and I had no idea what was really happening or how long I would survive. This was not the retirement that my second husband and I had recently planned and I felt horrified for my wider family, who had already suffered so much loss through the destructiveness of cancer amongst many relatives. At that moment there appeared to be absolutely no hope for any of us...

I spent several days in hospital until I stabilised. Upon being sent home I quickly discovered that I had lost some of my faculties. I could read but not write any letters or numbers. I could answer challenging questions on quiz shows but couldn't find where the longstanding switch for the bathroom light was situated. My conversations, and general understanding, could be either coherent or confused, alternating between the two very swiftly.

All hope was not lost, however. I was quickly sent back to the Churchill Hospital, where a team of oncologists, fully aware of my history, had devised a program of medical interventions that would potentially improve the quality of my life and hopefully extend it too. It was decided that I would be put on a course of targeted gene therapy drugs (Binimetinib and Encorafenib). These work by blocking the proteins that cancer cells give off and shrinking tumors in the process, whilst leaving healthy tissue in the vicinity alone.

So, almost six months down the line how hopeful are things? My mental faculties have returned, and I can now write, enjoy both number and word puzzles and most importantly laugh and chat again with those I care about. Nevertheless, side-effects from the medication have been numerous, often unpleasant and it feels like I have experienced most of those listed on the information leaflets that come with the drugs. Things vary from day-to-day according to the latest problems to emerge; some are reasonable and others awful, but I am learning to manage many of the issues more successfully as time goes on with the help of the dedicated oncology team.

Recent scans have shown some good news though, if only temporarily; some tumours have shrunk or become inactive while others have even disappeared. My sense of hope wavers from day to day, according to how well I feel but I don't feel as despondent as I formerly did. Hope for me now means being able to do small and pleasurable things: visiting friends for a meal, staring at the sea, a drive over Dartmoor on a clear day. However, perhaps most importantly, Hope—quite coincidentally—is the name of our three-year-old granddaughter so it is a word that always injects positivity into our everyday vocabulary.

Anna Wheeler

Anna wrote her story in spring 2022. She learned to cope with many of the side effects of her medication, mainly by changing to a 'Low FODMAP' diet and although we knew that her condition was terminal, her improved quality of life made the situation more manageable. However, in August 2022 her condition deteriorated rapidly due, we later found out, to further bleeds on the brain, and she was admitted to the local hospice for palliative care.

The large turnout for her funeral was testament to the impact she'd made on so many people in her career as a music teacher, her playing in various music groups, her community work, and the friends she'd made in so many other circles.

Anna was a massive Beatles fan and passed at the age of sixty-four so maybe it is fitting that, when she played a decaying and neglected piano in Pyramiden in the Arctic a few years earlier, and her rendition of 'When I'm sixty-four' was cut short due to the piano missing several vital parts, she laughed and said, *"I've run out of chords."*

Anna may have run out of chords but her music lives on in all she touched.

David Wheeler & Jenny Green
October 2022

A Hand Full of Hope

IT WAS 2012 AND I WAS PREPARING TO GET MARRIED BACK HOME IN SCOTLAND, while living and working in England. My partner had proposed to me on my thirtieth birthday and we planned to wed less than twelve months later.

My physical fitness peaked, naturally wanting to look my best for the big day, and I was physically feeling great. At the same time, I also felt constantly tired and was no doubt physically and mentally pushing myself too hard. The wedding day was all I had hoped for and we returned to England a week later.

When I was seventeen, I decided to pursue a career in nursing and loved my first year at university. One of the first things we were taught was the importance of self-examination which included how to check our breasts for any signs of cancer. While I changed my career to become a psychologist, that training stayed with me for all those years and I continued to carry out monthly checks. When I returned home from our honeymoon in Scotland I realised I hadn't checked myself for a couple of months and did so that night. I could feel a hard, gritty lump above my breast and I knew it didn't feel right.

The next day I phoned my GP and explained that I had found a lump. After a few days I attended my GP appointment and, following an examination, was assured that it didn't feel sinister but I would be referred to the community hospital for an oncologist to confirm that all was okay.

I remember going into the hospital where I met the nurse and the oncologist who were laughing and joking with another patient; they seemed so nice and caring and I was immediately put at ease.

The oncologist invited me into the room and tried to reassure me while looking through the referral notes. As soon as the physical examination started the atmosphere suddenly changed. The oncologist asked the nurse for a test tube and scalpel and took a biopsy of the lump—without any local anaesthetic—immediately raising concerns. At that moment, I regretted attending the appointment with no one by my side for support.

The oncologist sat me down and started writing on a piece of paper which had a diagram of a human body on it. He took his pen out and put a large circle around the area where he had removed the sample and wrote four times, 'URGENT'. He said he didn't have any appointments at his next clinic, which was in two days' time, but told me to turn up anyway with the piece of paper and inform the receptionist that I had to be seen that day.

I looked at him and said, *"So what you're telling me is that I've probably got cancer"*. He tried to reassure me by saying *"It's probably nothing,"* but by this time I could see that he was trying, and failing, to reassure me.

I remember trying to stay composed but could feel my body shaking and had a sensation of pins and needles throughout my body as I walked out of the room. I knew deep down that this wasn't looking positive.

My mum and dad were due to come down from Scotland for a visit on the same day I was going into hospital. I told them the evening before that I was going into hospital for a check-up and that there was nothing to worry about. It seemed awful not telling them at the time, but I suppose I wanted to protect them until I knew what I was dealing with.

The next day I went to the hospital with my husband by my side and they carried out an ultrasound, took another biopsy and some blood samples.

I sat outside in the waiting room, for what felt like hours, waiting on the outcome of all the tests. The waiting was the worst part. Deep down I knew it was cancer and although I'm not usually an anxious person, I was rocking forwards and backwards with my husband trying to calm me down. I was finally called in to see the oncologist. He said that they didn't have all the test results back but was 99.9 per cent sure it was cancer.

Nothing can prepare you for that moment.

I asked him if I was going to die, and he said that I might. It felt like an out of body experience and without thinking too much about it, I asked how long I had to live. He responded, *"How long is a piece of string?"* and I remember the wave of fear that swept through me. I can't remember much more about what happened after that response other than the oncologist apologising for being terrible at breaking bad news as he could never find the right words to say. He was being honest and I respected him for that.

I had to stay for other tests to prepare me for an operation to remove lymph nodes which would determine if the cancer had started to spread; it all seemed so surreal.

My parents called while I was in hospital asking when I would arrive back at my home. They had arrived in England that afternoon. I answered and said I was still waiting to be seen by the oncologist. I had already received the devastating news, but I couldn't tell them over the phone. When I finally arrived home and they opened the door to me, my mum just knew something wasn't right. I sat down with my parents and shared my news with them. Mum just went numb; she couldn't speak and left the room to cry. I tried to reassure them both and as dad tried to speak his voice broke. I had never seen my dad cry before. Dad has always been this solid, dependable rock in our lives, and this was the first time he felt completely helpless— they both did—as they knew this was one thing they couldn't fix.

I always thought it was worse for my family, as they had no control over the situation. My parents were always there to mend my physical scrapes and bruises, comfort me when I didn't achieve as well as I had hoped during my exams, but they were helpless for the first time as they couldn't take away the cancer. It was distressing to see them so upset. Looking back now, I hope they know how amazing they were through my cancer journey.

I returned to the hospital two weeks before Christmas to meet my surgeon and discuss my mastectomy and lymph node biopsy. Whilst we sat in his office he flicked through his diary, saying how busy he was and how he would struggle to fit me in any time soon. There was no sense of urgency or realisation that I was someone who had just received devastating, life-changing news and was waiting for a date to remove cancer that was potentially going to kill me. I was booked in for February and I left the meeting feeling distraught.

My husband could see that I had started to lose some hope and we agreed that we would seek private treatment so that I could receive better care. We didn't have much money, having just paid for our wedding and having recently finished university with new jobs that didn't pay very well, but we both agreed that the priority was getting surgery and treatment as soon as possible.

I will never know if what happened next was fate, destiny, divine intervention, or pure luck, but the next day I went into work to see my boss to discuss handing over my workload and taking time off. A close colleague had heard the news from my boss that morning. She walked up to me, hugged me and we both cried. She handed me a note with her husband's mobile number on it. He was the head of breast oncology at another hospital and was going to take me on as his patient. A moment in my life I will never forget.

Things then moved very quickly, and hope returned as I was quickly taken into the other hospital a few days later. I met my new oncologist who discussed my care plan. He then introduced me to my surgeon who booked me in for a lymph node biopsy and mastectomy, making sure I would be out of hospital in time to travel back to Scotland for Christmas to be with my family. The care and consideration were more than I could have hoped for.

My oncologist asked me if I was the type of person that just wanted to know if I'd be okay, or if I wanted all the information about my prognosis, treatments and outlook.

As a psychologist and health researcher, I spent most of my time reviewing or analysing health data and I asked for all the reports and articles that were available on my type of cancer—including survival rates. I needed to build a picture of what I was dealing with and to start taking back some control of my life.

After receiving the results of the type of cancer I had—stage two, grade three and HER-2 positive—and the realisation that it was quite an aggressive cancer which had started to spread to one of my lymph nodes, the oncologist decided that I should also have chemotherapy and radiotherapy. Despite having an aggressive cancer, my prognosis was good thanks to advances in cancer treatment. According to the statistics, I had a good chance of survival and being young would help me tolerate the gruesome treatment that lay ahead.

Cancer felt like a huge mountain I had to climb. Within a few days I had gone from feeling completely lost, with no hope, to being surrounded by support and a pretty positive outlook. I was determined that I would conquer that mountain.

I asked my husband to shave my hair off not long after I started treatment; my hair has always been very precious to me, and I couldn't bear watching it fall out. Shaving it off gave me some control back over my life and we made the experience fun and positive—there were laughs while we shaved my hair off, there were no tears. Looking back, there were a lot of laughs during treatment because I refused to feel sorry for myself and I was determined to make the best out of a horrific situation.

I'm a very positive person and people rarely see me being upset or being negative but there were days and weeks where I felt I had no control about what the future would hold for me. Every day I would wake up and think about my cancer; first thing in the morning and last thing at night. No one prepares you for the impact a diagnosis has on you.

However, being told I had an excellent chance of survival gave me the hope and determination to get through all of my treatment; I just wanted to survive and knew that when this was all over, I would live my life to the fullest. That is exactly what I have done.

I was terrified at my first chemo session but the staff were so attentive and generous with their time. I had a number of infections as my immune system was being attacked by the treatment and I was rushed into hospital on two occasions, which was incredibly worrying for my family. The sessions continued when I was well enough and one day I sat opposite a woman in her seventies who had diamond rings covering her fingers. I couldn't take my eyes off her hands. Every finger had at least two beautiful rings, sparkling away in this place of darkness.

She saw me looking at the rings and asked if I wanted to know the story behind them. I said yes and she explained that when she was first diagnosed with cancer she was told her lifespan would be very limited. Her husband had bought her a diamond ring and promised to buy her a new one for every year she survived. Thanks to advances in cancer treatment, she had survived for more than two decades and had so many rings that her husband joked about killing her to save money. It's strange to think how you can laugh about cancer, but sometimes laughter is a great release, and her story gave me so much hope.

When I think of what hope meant to me, shortly after finishing my chemotherapy, I travelled to New Zealand and met my friend's mum at a wedding. She came over to me and gave me a huge hug and said she was diagnosed with breast cancer twenty years ago. Despite still having cancer when I met her, she had an amazing quality of life because of the treatment she received. Fast forward another 10 years and we are both still here. This gives me so much hope.

As an adult I hate climbing stairs, never mind hills, and 10 years on from my diagnosis I have just climbed Kilimanjaro to raise money for Cancer Research UK. I remember seeing my cancer battle as a mountain that was in the way of the rest of my life. I knew it was going to be tough and at times I would be scared, unsteady on my feet and fearful that I wouldn't make it to the top. I also knew that I was a fighter, and I was filled with hope;

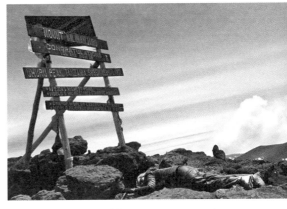

I had every intention of conquering that mountain so that I could continue on my path to a happy life and I did! Kilimanjaro was the toughest physical challenge of my life but also the most rewarding. I have been faced with climbing two mountains and I have conquered both. Cancer Research is why I am here and their continual advances in life-saving treatment gives me hope for a long, healthy and memorable life.

I want to give back that hope in any way I can.

Deborah Cairns

Fighting Together

MY LIFE CHANGED ON 29TH SEPTEMBER 2020 when I was admitted to Southampton General Hospital. I was working from home like most people during the pandemic and the previous day I had felt unwell, so I phoned my boss who'd told me to turn off my laptop and have a good sleep.

Despite trying that night, I couldn't sleep at all, as I had the most violent and uncontrollable hiccups all night long. Nothing I tried would stop them and by the morning I was desperate to phone the doctors.

Unable to get an appointment, I waited for a doctor to call me back. After explaining my symptoms, he advised me to go to A&E at the hospital to have some tests.

I called my wife to come home from work and asked her to take me to the hospital and I remember saying to her as we made our way out to the car, that I was dreading going in as I was afraid of what they might find. Though I really hoped it was nothing serious, I wasn't convincing myself.

I ended up being in hospital for nearly three weeks, as after various scans and tests they'd found a tumour blocking my stomach and I was given the news it looked like cancer.

My fears were realised.

The only option was to have an operation to remove the tumour so a right hemicolectomy was carried out, where a part of my large bowel was removed and the rest of my bowel was reconnected.

What followed were the longest three weeks of my life. My family weren't able to visit, I had a nasogastric tube permanently up my nose to feed me, and I found it increasingly hard to communicate using my phone as I kept losing my voice.

During my stay in hospital, I had several scans which unfortunately confirmed, along with the biopsy done on the twenty-four lymph nodes they had removed, that the cancer had spread to my lymph system.

As a result my oncologist started me on a course of chemotherapy immediately and discussed with me whether I would be able to pay for a new immunotherapy drug called Avastin which he thought I could react well to, but which wasn't available on the NHS.

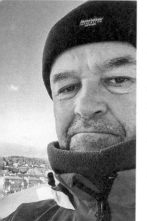

I set up a crowdfunding page hoping that people would help to cover this cost, which we couldn't, and was completely overwhelmed when nearly two-hundred people contributed, raising over £5,000, which meant I could have the treatment.

After 12 sessions of chemotherapy and immunotherapy, the last one being on 23 April 2021, I was sent for a scan and blood test. To my relief the results showed no new cancer growth and the oncologist said he'd monitor my bloods every three months with a new scan every six months.

Fast forward to May 2022 and my latest scan results continue to show no new cancer growth and when I asked my oncologist if he would describe my scan now as showing No Evidence Detected of cancer (NED), he replied by saying in his opinion that would accurately describe my current situation.

Considering when I asked him for my prognosis in January 2021 he told me he thought my life expectancy at that point was two years, to now be showing on scans as NED is a real story of hope for everyone.

During my treatment I was particularly pleased to speak to the MacMillan financial support team, who were fantastic at arranging my Personal Independence Payment (PIP) and a blue badge for parking. My support contact there helped me to fill in the forms I needed and they got a lot of items sorted, which took a lot of stress away.

My local hospital has a new Maggie's centre which opened as I started my treatment. I went in to meet the team and they explained what they did to support patients and we started with online therapy sessions, due to Covid. They introduced me to relaxation and exercise sessions, and importantly I got to meet other cancer patients, all with different types of cancer and stages.

I still go to the monthly living with cancer group at Maggie's,—this is a closed group that you have to be invited to,—and a small group of us attend and we support each other. We have built up a great relationship with each other, and we know what we've all been through, and this give us all hope, which we get from each other.

Our small group have realised that we don't need to battle this on our own, and we all have different experiences which we share with each other, and we have seen the positive impact this has, especially on new members.

It felt as if we make a difference to each other, by giving support and hope and it's so important to realise you're not alone.

When I was first diagnosed, I thought about things we wanted to do in the potential time available and my wife and I wanted to see the Northern Lights, which we have always dreamed about. We hoped that we could see St Elmo's Fire and we are now doing this in a few months' time on a cruise to the Arctic Circle. When we booked it, I didn't know what would happen with my cancer. I contacted my oncologist to ask if I was going to be okay to go on the cruise and he said if you're going to do it, do it this year. Thankfully things have changed, and he is now more positive.

I try to keep active every day by walking (setting a 10,000 steps a day target), I drink green tea, filtered water and have as much fruit and veg in my diet as possible. I have also cut back on eating red meat as well, preferring chicken and fish options instead.

I try to surround myself with positivity where I can, either by watching/listening to programmes on the TV/radio where there's a positive feel to the discussions, Chris Evans' Breakfast Show on Virgin Radio is an example. An important activity for me is spending time with my two young grandsons, who are so full of joy and mischief. I get quite teary when I think of the time I would have missed with them, if the treatment wasn't successful.

My hope comes from different places, and talking to other cancer patients not only gives me hope, but gives hope to them.

Keith Soley

Hope is Constant

ITHINK I **ALWAYS WANTED TO BE A NURSE.** I like helping people and even as a child I liked helping people. I was about eight or nine and I remember someone falling in the street and skinning their knee and, even although I didn't know them, I thought I needed to help and make them feel better. I suppose I've always had it in my blood.

When I was sixteen, I did a pre-nursing course after leaving school. The course prepared me for nursing and gave me an insight into the role by spending time at various local hospitals. I quickly learned that nursing was the profession I wanted to join. I then worked at a care of the elderly hospital as a nursing auxiliary. This gave me a great experience and I soon realised that being a nurse involved talking to the patients, trying to put them at their ease, letting them and their families know what was going to happen and supporting and caring for them throughout their time in hospital.

I loved the variety of work assisting the nurses and doctors and I would look forward to chatting to the patients and hearing about their life experiences and the things that were important to them.

In 1982 I started my nurse training, travelling to various hospitals and spending time in many areas covering general medicine, surgical, paediatrics and psychiatry. I really enjoyed the training as I got more experience in many different aspects of nursing.

Once qualified I worked in various medical wards with patients who had respiratory, gastroenterology and cardiac problems and where some of the patients had serious conditions that required one-to-one nursing. I enjoyed the fast pace of these wards, and I gained much experience from the senior nurses, doctors and the patients themselves.

As a nurse you knew that part of your job would involve dealing with the death of patients. In my nurse training we discussed the subject of death but there was limited support for nursing staff in the 1970s and no formal training on how to support the family, or how we were supposed to cope with the death of patients ourselves.

You learned how to cope with help from your senior colleagues and it is an element of study which has greatly improved over the years. The best advice I got from a colleague was to treat a person who had died as if they were still living, referring to them in the present tense. This helped me greatly and allowed me to nurse them with the same compassion in death as I had given them in life. You learned to cope with death as time went by, but it was always hard to accept.

I took some time off to have a family and then I returned to join a pool of medical nurses when my children were at school. As an experienced nurse I did short shifts in various departments, wherever help was needed. I was already known by the senior staff in the hospital and with my experience I was trusted to work with all patients.

During this time, I noticed that whilst the level of care was very high, I found myself wanting to give more time to the patients. In the wards, staff were very busy, and giving the additional time to chat with the patients during their difficult journey was limited, and this upset me. One area where I found this particularly prevalent was when nursing cancer patients.

This drew me to oncology where I knew I could give patients the additional time I wanted to.

After discussions with senior management, I had a secondment in the oncology unit which I found very rewarding. I felt I had more time to dedicate to the patients and when a post became available in the oncology unit I applied and was delighted to be successful in my application.

I had to do further degree course modules to be able to work in oncology which was a very specialised unit. These modules covered chemotherapy administration, cannulation, the completion of treatment packs, psychology and other topics as required.

We also had training on how to support the patients and how to deal with mental health issues during the patient's cancer journey. These courses were very valuable and, coupled with my medical experience and the support I gained from senior colleagues, helped me immensely.

We had an excellent senior manager in the oncology centre who always encouraged and supported us to do courses and whilst there was a lot of studying, this made me a better nurse and the patients benefited greatly.

It was not until I was doing the job, and gaining further experience working with other oncology staff, that I learned how to work with the patients on a personal level.

You didn't always have the same time in general wards to build a personal relationship with the patients, and you didn't always have enough time to discuss non-medical issues. In oncology you had more time to speak to people and build a personal relationship. Once you had built that relationship, everyone benefited.

When patients arrived for the first time in the oncology unit, as to be expected, they were very apprehensive, and some were frightened.

If a patient arrived frightened, I tried to put myself into their situation and my initial role was to calm them by talking, explaining their treatment as simply as possible and, above all else, by listening.

There were so many questions they had, and you had to answer them as best you could: what was going to happen, what treatment were they getting, what could be the side effects, and would it work?

This is when hope came in, when you managed to build up a relationship with the patient and when you spoke with them about everyday things, rather than constantly focusing on medical aspects.

This is when they would open up and say what was bothering them. Often the patient found the information so overwhelming that they were unable to absorb what was being said. However, they were encouraged to bring a friend or family member with them when they came for treatment, even just to hold their hand when the cannula was going in. It also helped to reinforce the details of the treatment to both people knowing that their friend or family member were more likely to retain the information we passed on to them.

I was aware that this changed during Covid and even though I had retired by then, I often thought about the patient who couldn't take anyone with them and how apprehensive they might have felt.

As a nurse I always strove to ensure that the patient's safety was paramount and that no harm would come to them.

I was trained to deal with the medical side of the patient's treatment and I was also trained to look out for patients who needed additional support and refer them to other multidisciplinary teams such as cancer support, psychology services and many other support teams.

As an oncology nurse we were trained to not give patients false or unrealistic hope. This was incredibly important. It was in our nature to say, *"don't worry"* and *"everything will be fine"*, but as an oncology nurse you couldn't say that.

Sometimes a conversation, and listening to them, was the best medicine.

In the oncology unit we were advised not to be emotional in front of the patient and their family if the patient had received bad news, but as a small nursing team we would get together to support each other during difficult times which always helped.

Being a good oncology nurse is about having a positive attitude, finding methods to cope during the difficult times and honouring the patient and their family who fought until the end.

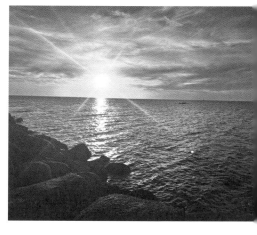

In time the patients got to know all the staff and we built a personal relationship during their treatment. Sometimes patients would build a stronger bond with a specific nurse, and they would get upset if that nurse was not on shift, nevertheless, we would do our best to meet their needs.

One of the best parts of being an oncology nurse was seeing patients build a bond with each other throughout their treatment. People that had never met each other before, suddenly had a unique shared experience and could become lifelong friends and give each other hope.

There was always hope at the different stages of a patient's cancer journey. Patients would get the shock of their diagnosis, but hope would take the form of hoping the treatment would work, and perhaps trials would be available for new treatments and that they would have more time with friends and family.

When we found out nothing had worked for patients who were treated with multiple drugs and/or trials, hope transitioned from hoping that the treatment would work to hoping that palliative care would meet their and their family's needs.

Hope that they would be pain-free, that they would be alert enough for their family to visit, that they would be able to say their goodbyes, and hoping that they would not be frightened.

When I first started as an oncology nurse, I hoped everyone would survive, but I knew that this wasn't realistic. Throughout my training and career, we were always aware of new research, drug developments and trials. We were very aware that hope was being developed in the oncology setting and I certainly saw more and more people survive cancer and I am still amazed at the advancements in such a short space of time.

Once I had retired, I would still meet patients on the street or in a shop and they would smile and stop for a chat and share a bit, or a lot, of their story post-treatment. This was the best job satisfaction I could have had, hearing about their success and I was always so humbled that they wanted to share it with me.

When I think about hope and the time I spent with patients, their families, and friends, I truly believe that hope is constant, it just takes on different forms.

Anon

You Don't Know How I Feel

I **WAS DIAGNOSED WITH MELANOMA CANCER IN AUGUST 2018.** There was a mole on the side of my face; I didn't pay much attention to it as it had been there for a long time. My daughter had come home for a visit from London, and said I should get the mole checked out as it looked different to the last time she had seen it.

I hadn't noticed any change, so I took her advice and I went to my GP who referred me to the dermatology clinic. Not thinking it was anything serious, I went on my own and was surprised when they removed part of it and said it would be tested. They would get in touch once the results came back.

The wait isn't very nice and like most people, I hoped it wasn't cancerous. When the results came back, I was told the mole was cancerous, and I would need surgery to remove it and the surrounding skin. As it was on my face I was quite concerned at the scar it would leave, but my plastic surgeon did a fantastic job and it was hardly noticeable.

My after-care was a check-up every three months and I felt confident this had now been dealt with.

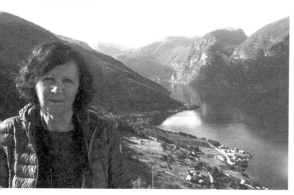

Life returned to normal until I discovered a small lump in my neck 18 months later, which was just at the start of the first Covid lockdown. It turned out that my melanoma had spread to the lymph nodes in my neck. This was a very traumatic time as I had to attend appointments and various scans on my own, plus receiving bad and good news over the phone, rather than face-to-face.

In June 2020 I had neck surgery to remove forty-six lymph nodes. Thankfully the surgery was successful and there were only two nodes affected by melanoma. This was good news and my physical recovery from the surgery was uneventful.

However, the mental scars of being in hospital for a number of days during Covid lockdown, with no visitors, started to build.

I was offered a year's course of immunotherapy as a preventive measure, and I took up the opportunity. This was also pretty much straightforward, and I suffered very few side effects.

It was a very lonely and scary experience having treatment in the hospital every four weeks. I felt guilty for being relatively well when those around me in the ward seemed much more ill. I felt I should be grateful for escaping the trauma of the side effects—but I didn't feel that way.

I was scared that it would be me one day.

However, just as I neared the end of my treatment my partner was diagnosed with colon cancer and he undertook major surgery and follow-up preventive chemotherapy and I couldn't really think about myself at that time.

It wasn't until I finished my treatment that I realised what a toll these experiences had taken on my mental health. When I think about hope during that period, it could be elusive. It comes and goes at different points. I always had hope, whether it was evident to other people, I don't know.

My friends and family were all very happy and congratulated me on staying the course and I know that I should have felt that way too, but I didn't. I couldn't understand why I felt the way I did and blamed myself for not feeling happy. I didn't want to talk about how I felt, thinking that others would think I was weak or something similar.

I tried to avoid situations where I might be asked how I was and if they did, I just said, *"I'm doing fine"*, knowing full well I wasn't. I did have a couple of friends and family members that I could talk to, and I felt they understood—especially those who had had similar experiences. I just didn't feel right in my own mind, and I found it difficult to talk to people as I thought people would expect me to get on with my life and put it all behind me.

What has she got to complain about?

I became very sensitive to what people were saying and often picked up on what could be thought of as inappropriate remarks. I also became very sensitive to the fact that some people didn't know what to say when I talked about how I was feeling.

By chance I spoke with someone from Maggie's Centre, and that's when I realised it is perfectly normal to feel like this after you finish treatment.

It was a real light bulb moment for me. I had some counselling and took part in a course run by the centre with other cancer patients. It's taken a while for me to come to terms with what I have been through but I'm getting there. My partner and I are getting our fitness back and we are planning to run 10k in the Edinburgh Marathon next year to raise money for charities that have helped both of us through our journey.

I think it's important to share stories about our cancer experiences with others, as it is a very scary time. My neighbour is now a close friend as she shared her cancer journey with me, which I hadn't been aware of. She understood.

It's difficult when you are going through treatment to think about the future when all you are thinking about is your next treatment, appointment, or scan. I found that hope comes along in little snippets. It wasn't the great big things like *"I hope I don't die"*, it's hoping each stage is positive. The next oncology meeting, my biopsy, hoping the surgery doesn't leave too visible a scar, and that I get good scan and x-ray results.

I have learned that hope can also be very elusive. It hovers about in the background and pops its head up, often when you least expect it. Recently I have fond myself thinking about the future—what will I buy for Christmas presents, will I visit my brother in America next year? That's hope telling me there is some!

I am sure this story will chime with a lot of people and I hope it brings some comfort, however small.

Fiona

The Journey by Keith 'Rin' Ryan

The boatman casts the bowline, once so tight,
From the shore into the night
My keel is still holding fast
The journey to the sea
may be my last

The Ettrick flows into the sea
They change its name, it's you, it's me
The rain has fallen to its fate,
Gathered now, it's in full spate

Running with the current flow,
Against the tide you cannot go.
The rudder it is all we have
To steer the boat, its journey cast

The Ettrick flows into the sea
They change its name, it's you, it's me
Bonnie, bonnie Ettrick side,
Into her depths I musn't slide

Bow to stern we must relearn
to live the life, that we yearn
Live, love and turn
New and old, precious gold

The Ettrick flows into the sea
They change its name, it's you, it's me
Throughout history it's cut the hill,
Over the cauld and past the mill

Hidden rocks, as we slide
On the journey to the tide,
We'll find an eddy, wait and see
They change its name, it's you,
IT'S ME.

Keith Ryan

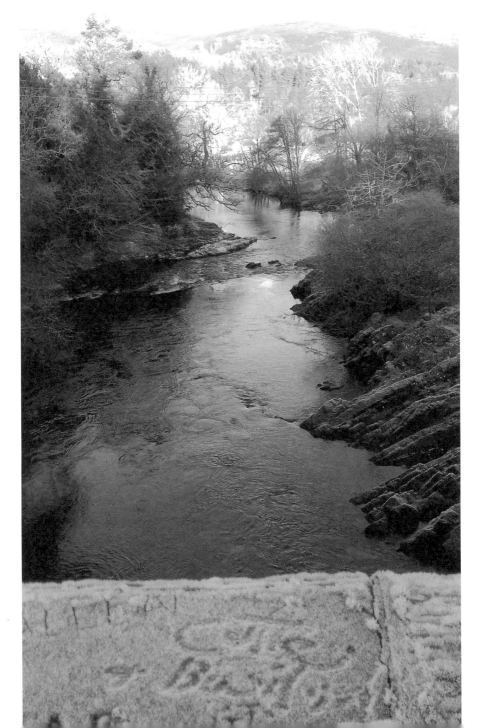

Thirty Years After...

IT WAS EXPLAINED IN THE PINK BOOKLET on reconstruction that the new breast would not look quite like your own (paraphrasing) but more like a young woman's. The other breast could be matched later, if you chose, with cosmetic surgery. Well, that was certainly worth considering—and all on the NHS. Not for the first time, I was grateful to have these options. On the one hand, I thought flippantly, what's not to like? In truth, the loss of a breast was a fearful prospect.

I'd had surgery on the same breast twelve years before, when I was quite young: removal of a cancerous tumour which appeared to be the size of a pea, and a small section around it. The cancer (malignant neoplasm) had been caught early. I'd found the tiny lump myself, persisting albeit slightly discouraged by the instruction to 'come back and see him (the GP) if it got any larger'. Fortunately for me, I did go back, though I honestly could not tell if it had grown; I only knew it was definitely still there. Testing of lymph nodes after my lumpectomy showed the cancer hadn't spread. I'd then gone as an outpatient for a five-week course of radiotherapy, which was pretty straightforward. There had been some swelling and redness (like sunburn) as expected and I'd been advised to avoid potential infection from smoke-filled atmospheres. I was a musician and this was long before the smoking ban. But I'd continued playing and performing with the band, in fact it had felt essential to my sense of identity and a perfect antidote! I was fairly fit, as noted by fellow radiotherapy patients who would see me striding away from these appointments on my way across the city.

Reading up on free radicals and other factors which contribute to cancer, I made some changes to my diet, moved into a new flat with some friends and felt hopeful. For several years afterwards I was reassured by regular mammograms as well as annual physical check-ups from a dedicated female doctor at the hospital. Each time, I was good to go. It seemed I had nothing further to worry about.

I was in the process of relocating some distance away, when I had to decide what to do about the final examination. After twelve years, I was considered in the clear. I could, if I wished, opt out of the last check-up... it was up to me. I had just one niggling concern: a very small lump which had reappeared in almost exactly the same place as before. I had felt something on my scar some months previously, and had mentioned it at the last check-up. At the time, it was thought this was part of the scar tissue from the old surgery, which I accepted.

The move went ahead as planned. However, in light of this miniature lump, and probably with a doctor's referral letter (though the details are hazy), I attended the large hospital in my new district for what, I assumed, would be my very last check-up. I was impressed to hear they would use a blood test which could reveal the presence of breast cancer. It seemed miraculous to be able to detect cancer in this way! Even so, I was so confident I was fine that I told my partner, Rin, he needn't come in with me to hear the result. (He waited in the nearby canteen all the same.) I sat facing a doctor and a specialist nurse, fully expecting to hear my test was negative.

But no.

I was stunned to the core to be told the cancer had come back. In a daze, I asked for my partner to be called, while the doctor expressed surprise that I was so completely unprepared for this possibility. Rin promptly joined me to hear the news. I'd need to have a mastectomy. I was aghast. Couldn't I just have the lump removed, as before? As the proposed path of my treatment was outlined, it was explained that had that first occurrence of cancer been diagnosed nowadays, they would have recommended a mastectomy there and then (rather than the lumpectomy plus the course of radiotherapy I'd received.) More was now known about breast cancers and the most effective ways to treat them. I began to understand there are many different types of breast cancer, for which treatments can vary. Once again, the prompt detection was in my favour.

Things moved like lightning from that point, a blur of activity. I continued working for a short while as a professional fund-raiser for various charities, including a little-known cancer charity (for which I had to be the most ardent fund-raiser on the team!) fitting this around the next scan or appointment. I scoured all the information I was given on mastectomy, what it meant, how a reconstruction might look. I stole myself to break the news to my parents. I'd never told my mother about the first instance of cancer and had sworn my father to secrecy, as mum had been unwell in hospital and I hadn't wanted to worry her. I needed to come clean. After the initial shock, my distressed parents had trouble understanding the need for a mastectomy. I convinced them this was on the basis of solid medical advice, non-negotiable.

Late on the night before my mastectomy, I crept into the loos of the old Victorian breast-cancer ward to draw and write in my journal. I admit to feeling a bit sorry for myself. I was soon to realise that some women on the ward had cancers which were more advanced. I was saddened to hear one lady had yet to tell her children, a painful dilemma for her. I was sure they would want to know, as had my parents, and wondered how isolated she must feel. Thinking back to chats with these lovely ladies on that ward, I am struck by their openness and complete lack of self pity. Although I could not fully grasp the enormity of what some of them may be facing, it put my case into sharp focus: I was one of the lucky ones. It was the overriding theme which stayed with me.

And hope? It was there, in the good friends and family who rallied round and buoyed me up with kind messages and gifts for my hospital stay. My partner's sister Ann and family, so supportive; his brother Chris, generously putting us up for as long as we needed. Lou, my sister, and my friend Roxana, each travelling great distances to see me. Above all, my partner Rin, by my side always.

We hoped—were certain, even—I would survive. I occasionally ask myself where that certainty came from? Probably the fact that I was youngish, early forties, and so far relatively untouched by loss. Or at least, the sort that rocks your foundations.

The whole raft of support, information and advice available at the hospital inspired confidence. And my kind specialist cancer-care nurse—a gem. One regret is that I didn't embrace the opportunity she offered, which was to join a network of other breast cancer patients and survivors, listening to and sharing with those going through the same. Perhaps

I wanted to leave this behind me… or I felt inadequate, fearing I'd say 'the wrong thing'—is there a 'right thing'?—in such a maze, through which our paths follow for a time a similar course, then diverge; or intersect and occasionally reconnect somewhere down the line.

This life-threatening disease affects so many women, and men, of all ages and walks of life. I'm incredibly thankful for my early diagnoses. In both cases I found evidence of the tumour myself: tiny, the size of a pea. So I always say, check yourself regularly, don't rely solely on mammograms as they don't catch all signs of cancer. Know your body and don't hesitate to get anything unusual or worrying investigated. Time is of the essence.

Some months after the mastectomy, I went ahead with a breast reconstruction under an excellent reconstructive surgeon at the same hospital. He took immense time and care and, together with his wonderful personal secretary, gave me hope I would appear—and feel—restored and whole again.

After recovering from the successful, complex reconstruction operation, I bought a breast cancer t-shirt to celebrate. 'GORGEOUS' emblazoned in pink on black with a pink ribbon, which I proudly wore as I left.

Here I still am, thirty-odd years after that first diagnosis, nearing twenty since the second. I'm acutely aware that my life has been saved—when others have not. I still wonder at how arbitrary that seems and am sure I'm not alone.

Finally, I want to offer hope and say to anyone diagnosed with breast cancer: stay positive, very many of us have treatment and do survive.

Cate
For Rin

Hope is a Gift to Each Other

I FELL INTO THE PHARMACEUTICAL INDUSTRY IF I'M HONEST. I wasn't aware of the industry and my parents had always encouraged my sister and I to do what we were passionate about. I wanted to study environmental science and after getting the grades I needed, I went to Kings College London. I loved it.

After graduation, my objective was to get a job in science, earn some money and to stay in London, which I had fallen in love with.

After a few temp jobs, and applying for jobs in science, I started at my current company as an entry level administrative assistant, in order to get my 'foot in the door'.

I started to work on clinical trials in the 1990s, involved in filing case notes and managing the study reports, and I found myself working on treatments for viruses, specifically HIV.

Our company was developing drugs in this field, and as HIV is an auto-immune disease, I got to know a lot about the human immune system. Study of viruses started to fascinate me and there was a lot of research going on in the field of virology to combat HIV, which had very limited treatment options for patients at that point.

At that time, I was vaguely aware of the options for cancer treatment, which were limited to radiotherapy or chemotherapy. There was nothing else at that time and for those with cancers that wouldn't respond to either of those treatments, there were no other options.

I continued working on virology in research and development, monitoring clinical trials and project managing some of the research. I spent eighteen years in increasing positions of responsibility, working in research. I transitioned into other disease areas and, as immuno-oncology emerged (the stimulation of the immune system to treat cancer, improving on the immune system's natural ability to fight the disease), I started to work on the early development of those treatments.

People outside the pharma industry didn't really understand what I did in the early stages of my career, nor the impact we were having on people living with cancer. As hard as I tried, their faces would glaze over, and they would nod politely as I talked them through the various stages of drug development. But when I explain that at the heart of what we do is the hope that the drugs we develop might lead to cancer patients being cured, delaying the spread of the cancer, or patients generally spending more time with their friends and family, this resonated with them.

My work would expose me to the wonderful medical professionals working in the field of cancer, who were running clinical trials. Part of my job was to gather the key data and report on whether it was working—or not—and importantly I started to develop ways to track how those receiving the trials were feeling: how was their daily routine, their energy levels, ability to concentrate, general well-being and their mental health?

This focus on their well-being appeared to be revolutionary at the time, and it is now standard practice in trials.

I was blessed to form professional relationships with cancer charities that focused on people living with cancer and one of the people I met was Gill Nuttall from Melanoma UK. Melanoma UK are a patient advocacy charity that support people diagnosed and living with melanoma and non-melanoma skin cancer. Gill is inspiration in human form.

I moved from research and development to the strategy side of the business twelve years ago and have worked on our strategy and how to operationalise it in a more efficient way. How do we get science to our health care professionals quicker? How can we get our medicines to patients quicker? An example of how we collaborate, are advisory boards, to gain input from doctors, consultants, nurses and pharmacists from across the world. The purpose of an advisory board is to gain input on the trials we are running, and the trials we have planned for the future, so that we can ensure we are mapping to the needs of the patients and to those administrating the medicines.

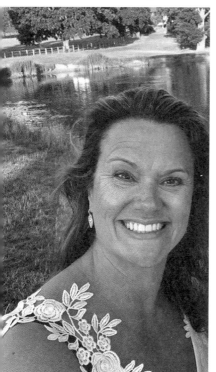

This is a very integrated approach and it's also vital that we include the cancer patient groups who have an amazing insight into what is required and, importantly, what will and won't work. They offer real life experience. Pharmaceutical companies are, quite rightly, not allowed to interact directly with patients and our window into their world is through cancer charities, our health care professionals and patient advocacy groups.

These groups make our strategy realistic, and an example might be how a drug needs to be taken, when it should be taken and how frequently. The patient groups will advise on the best way to ensure that the patient understands what to do, if they are self-administering, and how to make it easy for them to do so.

The drug development process is a huge undertaking and still takes us too long. My hope is that seeing how quickly scientists have developed Covid drugs and then had them administered, that we can learn lessons from that and get cancer and all other treatments to market much quicker.

The company I work for and the pharmaceutical industry strives to address the unmet medical needs of patients by investing in research and development. We exist to meet an unmet medical need and there is a cost for that, which is recovered through charging for the drugs which are proven to meet those needs. There are many drugs that don't become available, and that is the cost of research and development.

When I think about hope and what that means to me in my job, and I go back to those early HIV days and what the patients were going through, what all patients and their loved ones are going through and also, the limited treatments for cancer. There wasn't a lot of hope, compared to now.

Great leaps have been made in cancer treatment through immuno-oncology and other treatments, and we now see cancer as a fast-paced environment where hope is measured in increased survival rates, more patients being cured, and new revolutionary treatments for cancer.

We are now researching new treatments, and the oncology world is delivering targeted cancer medicines through personal customised treatments down to the level where treatment is specific to the patient's DNA.

Working on the development of new cancer treatments always brings hope that the treatment will work and will be approved, but the reality is that they don't all work and you know that there are patients who shared that hope, which was never realised.

It's incredibly hard when a drug doesn't work and the negative impact it has on patients and their families, and we have to move on to the next drug with the same hope. Like most people, I've lost friends, family, and colleagues to cancer and that is always with me in my job.

I get my hope from the amazing medical community we work with, the patients themselves who write to us, and the cancer patient charities.

I have a sign in my garden, which says *"To plant a garden, is to believe in tomorrow"*. I regularly look at that as I'm pruning the flowers or encouraging my tomato plants to grow. It's a line from Audrey Hepburn and to me, that is what hope is about, it's the belief in tomorrow. It's the belief in tomorrow that things are improving, things continue to change, and that keeps me going. I have heard patients say they look to pharmaceutical companies for hope, and I actually look to them for my hope.

My ultimate hope is that we cure cancer once and for all, and we are getting ever closer. It's not as quick as we want, but we are making faster progress.

Each week there are new developments and areas of hope and looking back to when I first started in the industry, the hope of curing cancer was never talked about.

Are we searching for a cure or a prevention for cancer? We're certainly looking for a cure and developing more ways to prevent cancer.

I believe that hope is a gift to each other.

Jo Cowler

I Took the Right Path

GROWING UP IN SOUTH AFRICA WITH A PALE COMPLEXION, I've always had moles and for the first forty years of my life they never presented any problems. When you live in a country that regularly breaches thirty degrees, you must be careful with your skin and whilst I had more moles than a farmer's field, I've taken great care to cover up and protect myself. My desire to keep out of the sun even stretched to seven years in the navy on submarines, just to avoid the sun.

Having travelled the world and lived in multiple countries, I found myself working in the Falkland Islands on a two-year contract in December 2019, taking my wife and my three-year-old daughter with me.

It was certainly a different climate to South Africa, Australia and Saudi Arabia and there wasn't much need for factor thirty let alone fifty. A few months into my contract I noticed a mole on the lower right part of my abdomen, which appeared to be growing, turning ugly and it had recently started to bleed.

My wife said I should get it checked out and so I booked an appointment with the GP, who having looked at it thought it was a twisted mole, but I wasn't convinced. Having a lot of moles, I was quite sure this one was more serious.

The GP advised me to keep monitoring it and to come back in two weeks time. I decided to go back earlier as it was continuing to bleed and I wasn't happy with how it looked or was behaving. On August 21st, I saw the GP who then asked a surgeon to come into the room and look at it, and the surgeon decided to operate the same day.

I wasn't mentally prepared for the surgery, and it certainly didn't go to plan. The plan was for the surgeon to cut the mole out and send it to the UK for analysis. As the surgeon was cutting the mole, after my side was anaesthetised, I could feel blood running down my side and I could hear it dripping onto the floor, no doubt building a pool. There was so much of it an orderly cautioned the surgeon about stepping in the blood on the floor, but he hadn't quite warned the surgeon in time, who slipped on my blood.

Once he had removed it, he showed me the mole and I was shocked to see how deep the root was. It looked like a baby carrot, and I knew this wasn't good. I returned to work, and I didn't feel great and then my wound got infected. Due to the sample having to be analysed in the UK, it took a month for the results to come back.

During that time, I managed to carry on working and I put it to the back of my mind. Cancer didn't even enter my thought process, as cancer happened to other people, didn't it?

When I walked into the GP surgery on September 21st to hear my results, I could see the worried look on his and the other staff members' faces.

I heard the word cancer, but it didn't sink in. I asked if the cancer was bad, and they said I would have to return to the UK for a wide area excision to remove the area around where the mole used to be. Through his explanation of the procedure, I was trying to remain positive and gather as much information as possible on the next steps and likely outcomes.

Looking back, as I explained this conversation with my wife, I can appreciate that the enormity of what was about to happen hadn't really hit home.

Within nine days, I was back in the UK, on my own, and within two days I spoke to my plastic surgeon for the first time. That night, sitting in my sparsely furnished holiday flat in the Scottish Borders, on my own, I cried. I'm not much of a crier, but all my fears and dark thoughts flooded out, and I filled the walls with my anguish.

I was fortunate enough to have both my grown-up children, Jason and Tarryn, living in Scotland and they would come and see me in my apartment, to help and offer me some comfort.

Soon the enormity of my situation had sunk in, and for the first time I was truly frightened. Sitting on my own, the dark thoughts were swirling around like a twister, and I needed to speak to someone that may be able to understand, and I quickly established a relationship with Macmillan, who I spoke to every week and these conversations helped me focus on the surgery ahead.

Having met the dermatologist at the hospital, we discussed another mole on my leg which started to grow and within two weeks the dermatologist had decided to remove it.

I still hadn't been for my wide area excision surgery, and it felt as if my body was starting to present multiple dangers at the same time, as he also decided to remove a mole on the side of my face. On the 19th of November 2020, I underwent surgery to remove the area surrounding the mole on my abdomen.

Once I came to, I suddenly realised that I had a pain under my arm, where they had removed lymph nodes to check if the cancer had spread. I was expecting them to have removed some from my groin, but the trace solution had shown a connection to my armpit.

This concerned me as I didn't know if it had spread to my groin as well, and shortly after this I was informed that the mole on my leg was cancerous and I would have to have to return for more surgery, two months later.

My wife and youngest daughter were still in the Falklands, and I was becoming increasingly worried at the path this was taking and being on my own. This put a great strain on my mental health.

I was so happy that my wife and daughter joined me in the UK on December 21st, but things did not turn out as I had hoped or planned. Three weeks after joining me in Scotland, we separated, and my wife left with my daughter to return to her home in Australia. I planned to visit them as soon as my surgery and recovery were completed in 2021, but then Covid struck again, and I was stuck on my own.

I prepared myself for my second surgery, which this time would involve removing lymph nodes from my groin and would restrict my mobility. Thankfully my grown-up daughter, Tarryn, was able to come down and give me a lift to and from the places I needed to go and provide much needed moral support. My son, Jason, was also always on hand.

I had the surgery, but I was left with a hematoma, which itself got infected. I was at my lowest ebb, as it seemed my body was still attacking me and combined with the impact of our separation and living on my own as Covid took a grip of the UK. Everything had conspired against me. What was there to live for?

I was in a desperate place mentally and as part of my recovery I would walk from my flat to the sea cliffs, which hugged the North Sea, and I found myself thinking, why don't I just keep walking when I get to the edge?

There was no hope. I had cancer in two places. It must surely be spreading, and I thought I would be dead within a year.

All hope had been taken from me.

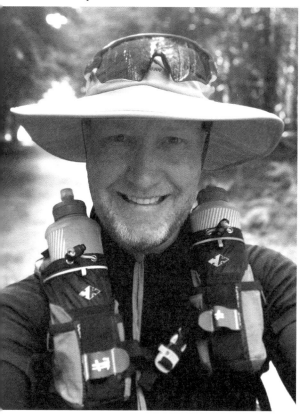

The morning of the 11th of February 2021, I had convinced myself to keep walking from the end of the cliff. I couldn't see a positive end to this. Before I set out for my final walk, I had been sifting through some paperwork and noticed a flyer for a melanoma charity, Melanoma UK. I had sent an email to the address on the flyer and got an immediate invitation to join a weekly Zoom call that evening with their community.

The thought of talking to and listening to people who had experienced the same as me, made me curious and I followed the cliff path that day, instead of veering off it.

That evening I shared my story with complete strangers, some of whom had been sharing their stories for weeks and had lesser and greater cancer diagnosis than me.

I let everything go on that call, and my new friends listened and let me unburden my physical and mental scars.

That very evening, my life was saved, and I found hope with this new community of melanoma survivors and thrivers. Having returned weekly for six weeks to these Zoom calls, I then got the news that the cancer from my leg had spread to my lymph nodes, and I know if I hadn't found my new friends, who welcomed me and assured me I was not alone, I would have walked off that cliff.

I'd formulated my plan, after speaking to the melanoma community, that I would progress with the treatment whether I was diagnosed with stage three or stage four cancer. They reassured me that there was a very good chance treatment would work.

My oncologist confirmed that there was no further spread, and my cancer was just in one lymph node, which gave me great hope and I knew then I would start the immunotherapy treatment and I would remain in the UK.

For the next thirteen months I would receive adjuvant treatment, to hopefully stop the cancer from spreading, and during that time I had another cancerous mole removed from my neck. I had put my whole trust in my oncology team.

Meanwhile, I had to deal with my employer in the Falklands trying to get rid of me, which involved legal consultation and more stress on top of my cancer treatment.

Looking back there was so much change in my life and whilst I consider myself to be a positive person, it's hard to articulate the depths you plummet to on this journey; dealing with cancer and its multiple baggage.

There is no doubt that talking and sharing my cancer journey with the Melanoma UK community, who had all walked the same cliff path as me, helped immensely and gave me hope, where there didn't appear to be any. The greatest gift I now have is helping others navigate their way along that path and helping them to understand that there is always hope.

Cancer has changed my life and now, following my treatment, I am cancer free and I'm confident in my hope for a long and happy life.

Daniel Wood

The Circle of Hope

IN THE SUMMER OF 1990, my husband Alistair, then aged fifty-three, began to have very debilitating health problems. In spite of having a range of tests over the next few months there was no positive diagnosis, though he became so exhausted that he had to stop work. In early December, the doctor decided a laparotomy was needed.

Then the hammer blow fell—it was cancer, non-Hodgkins lymphoma. There was a growth on the abdominal lymph gland, unsuspected, since he had actually put on some weight, not lost it, as was usual with cancer.

So there we were just after our Silver Wedding, where we had been planning all the things we wanted to do once we were retired, enjoying things we had never previously been able to afford. Now we faced a frightening dark tunnel, going nowhere. I remember sitting on the kitchen floor, hugging the dog and crying over the harsh treatment my beloved husband was facing and our shattered plans.

Strangely though, hope—the light at the end of the tunnel—came from Alistair himself. He had always tackled everything positively with energy and commitment and this was no different. From the moment of diagnosis his attitude was, *"It's treatable, so let's get on and get to remission. I have too much still to do and we're going to France in June."*

From then his attitude never changed. Although the initial chemotherapy proved too harsh, after being transferred to a regime of tablets he was soon back to work and we enjoyed our Easter visit to Wester Ross as usual. When it was time to go to France, with the chemo tablets packed, off we set for the ferry and the leisurely drive to our hotel, where he took the last of the tablets.

Life had returned to normal even before the all-clear. His positivity and determination had given us hope enough to do what we had already planned and actually doing it increased the hope, making us determined to keep looking forward, facing the future together.

Three years later, in 1994, a PSA test confirmed that he could soon develop prostate cancer. The choice was radical surgery or drug treatment which, if unsuccessful, might mean it was too late for surgery. He chose surgery for a faster recovery to get on with our lives again. With surgery in May that year and then France again in early July we realised that we, not the disease, were still in charge of our lives and could have a future.

Later that year, however, lymphoma returned. Past experience still gave us hope and the same chemotherapy enabled him to live fairly normally, with few side effects. Unfortunately, the consultant warned that the lymphoma would now return much sooner, with treatment less successful. Nevertheless, a new hope beckoned. The doctor knew that the professor of oncology at Bart's in London wanted 'guinea pigs' aged over fifty-five to undergo a relatively new treatment which could greatly extend life expectancy—a transplant of one's own bone marrow, harvested in remission and attacked aggressively in the lab, before being returned.

The doctor gave Alistair the next months of chemo to consider this but I knew that same day that Alistair would go for it. Was this determination, experience, and faith in his doctor or just plain hope? Neither of us doubted that it was the right choice. It would be a lie to say that I never secretly worried. There were times I lay awake at 2 am wondering what I would do if, in Bart's, a doctor said, *"I'm very sorry, but he is not going to make it."* But I never really lost the conviction that it would succeed and we would have more time together.

I went to Bart's with Alistair. A whole new experience, in which we shared every minute. Can one really enjoy any cancer journey? In some ways we did. The Professor believed that, if hygiene and cleaning were superb, all infections during treatment came from within the patient's body while their immune system was non-existent. So no isolation, only a restriction to hospital grounds, and the professor even visited on Saturday mornings—with his spaniel in tow! We were told to live as normal lives as possible, which undoubtedly helped us to focus on the future with hope and positivity.

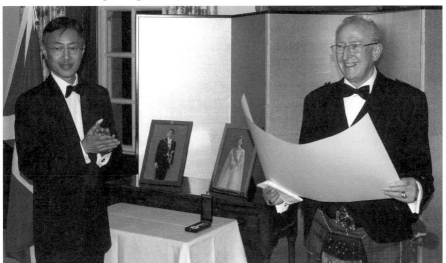

Alistair Simpson receiving the Order of the Rising Sun from the Japanese Consul General

I slept on a camp bed in Alistair's room, helped him dress, sat out in the grounds in the sun—even with a drip attached—and made gallons of chicken soup to tempt him to eat, the surplus going to the night staff! There was a fully stocked kitchen where patients and family could eat together and a washing machine and tumble drier. Alistair even had his entire desktop computer set up in his room. Even during this harsh treatment we lived fairly normally and made new friends, who are still in touch. I remember the little son of a patient who used to come and steal chocolate mousse from our fridge, if his mum forgot to buy it!

Finally, six weeks later, we were on our way home. With a few minor hiccups, Alistair's health improved and before long he was able to return to work. Checks were at first monthly, then three-monthly, then six, then a year, until, nine years later, he was told that he was so fit and well that there was no need for any further checks. So when age sixty came along we celebrated with a party at home—for twenty friends and family, self-catered by me, an event repeated every five years thereafter!

By then, we had used early retirement to start fulfilling our plans, mostly for travel. We visited places all over the world from Hawaii to Australia and New Zealand, from USA and Canada to Japan, while every year we went to France as usual, and latterly enjoyed European river cruises too.

For nearly eighteen years Alistair's health was excellent. Then he began to have heart problems and finally a liver tumour, so he then spent fourteen months in palliative care at home. Never once did he call for help from his Macmillan nurse—she made excuses to drop in—and after a short illness in hospital, he informed them he was going home. He arrived home on 27th March 2015 and was helped to bed where he died peacefully the next morning, with me and his younger son beside him, fifty years to the day from our engagement and four months before our Golden Wedding, for which he was still planning the party while in hospital.

Every day I still miss him but we had a wonderful life. He taught me so much about positivity and hope and I am so proud of him, especially for something unexpected. Six years after he died, World Wide Cancer Research, which funds ground-breaking research in universities worldwide, wrote up Alistair's story in their global newsletter. Within a month, they had received thousands in new donations and letters saying how inspiring the story was, with even a postcard for me! A legacy he knew nothing about.

We had just short of twenty five extra years together, and I can honestly say we had great fun. We saw our sons married and three granddaughters born. We lived our retirement to the full and cancer never determined our lives. In fact, the very sharing of every little bit of the journey, even appointments and clinics, meant that we never needed to discuss the disease. It was confined to these times only.

I believe, therefore, that hope is part of a circular process. A positive attitude and determination to meet the situation head-on makes hope automatic, and that hope helps maintain positivity. The real secret, for however long it takes, is sharing every bit of the journey with those closest, so that there is no need for cancer to run one's life. We never talked about cancer—we already shared the journey.

With every advance, therefore, in treatment or a new discovery or drug, someone benefits, just like Alistair. Well worth waiting and hoping!

Pat Simpson

The Cancer Club

NEVER SET OUT TO START A CANCER CHARITY, but then again, I never planned on getting cancer.

No one does and when it happens you place your trust in the white coats to guide you through the no man's land and minefields of cancer.

There is no manual, no textbook, no Ordnance Survey map to tell you where to go and what to avoid.

I started my bowel cancer journey in 2015. I started noticing my poo had some dark red blotches in it and it wasn't immediately obvious so I had to do a double-take. It didn't look or feel right so I decided to monitor it.

The night before I first noticed it, I was out with friends. I had a lovely steak and a probably a bit too much red wine, and I initially put it down to this.

It remained after a few days so I made a doctor's appointment. I saw a locum doctor who said we don't want to take chances so I'll book an endoscopy and colonoscopy, but don't worry too much it's probably nothing. As I had private medical insurance via work, I invoked this and got an appointment quite quickly.

I prepared for my colonoscopy which, for those that have not had one, understand it's not too pleasant and you have to stay close to a toilet the day before.

I was mildly sedated as the consultant worked the camera to have a good look at my bowel, which I was able to see as well. After a while he just calmly said, *"You've got cancer"*. The nurse was holding my hand and chatting to me quite casually, and then they took me into another room and left me on my own. It then started to sink in, slowly.

What do I tell my wife?

A while later the consultant came in and tried to reassure me by saying they had caught it early and surgery should take care of it. *"The surgeon will have it out in no time."*

I called my wife and asked her to collect me, as we had arranged, and I didn't feel scared or worried as I told her I had cancer, and they would remove it. I didn't think of hope at this point as I had complete faith in what I was being told.

It never occurred to me that I hadn't seen an oncologist at any point in this process, and I just put my trust in the team I was dealing with.

Within a four to six-week period I had gone from seeing the GP, being told I had cancer, to lying on the operating table.

The operation went successfully to remove the tumour. I was told there were clear margins, and I wouldn't need chemo, but there were complications with my bowel, and they had to give me an ileostomy bag. I couldn't eat properly, and I had to stay in hospital for two to three weeks until I got home.

I knew psychologically that the ileostomy could be reversed and whilst it took time to adjust, it didn't really get me down. It was inconvenient and weird, but it was temporary. The ileostomy was removed a few months later and they said I could go back to work.

It wasn't until years later I realised the absolute magnitude of what had happened, and I was very pleased to be told the cancer was Duke stage B, and there was no further need for anything else.

I passed all the information and invoices to my employer and then the fun began. It turned out that they hadn't put the insurance in place, which would leave me liable for all costs.

I formally raised this with them and it got rather messy. This turned out to be one of the most stressful periods in my life. If they had had everything in place, I would have been sorted. After a protracted period of time, many sleepless nights and immense worry we reached an agreement, and I left the company.

I was living a normal life by then and I had been one year clear of cancer, and I had secured another job, which I was enjoying.

In October 2016 I started to get a pain in my bum. I went back to see the surgeon who had operated and he thought it was scar tissue pain. The only way I could relieve the pain was by sitting in a hot bath, which would of course get quite cold after a while. The pain stretched from my rectum into my pelvic area, and I couldn't really put my finger on it, literally.

Given my history, I don't know why I wasn't referred to an oncologist.

I went for a PET scan and then saw the same surgeon again, and he delivered the news that the cancer had recurred and it was a local occurrence in my pelvic area. There was a growth touching the sacral nerve, near the base of my back, which was causing the acute pain.

Again he tried to reassure me that they had caught it early, but I was a bit wiser this time, and less likely to place my complete trust in his words of comfort.

When you are diagnosed with cancer one of the first pieces of advice you are given is 'don't start Googling'. There's a lot of medically verified information out there, but also some dangerous information. I wanted to know more about this cancer, so I did some online research. I found there was a less than twenty percent chance of this cancer happening. It felt like the beginning of a downward spiral and something we had experienced some years before when my mum had died of cancer and we had been through a constant stream of bad news about her condition.

With this diagnosis I was pretty low, even though I am a positive person, glass half-full with room for more, and the surgeon was still saying they could cure me.

At this point I was introduced to an oncologist, for the first time, and her advice was to pursue pelvic exenteration to remove my bladder, bowel, and prostate. It's hard to fully understand how big this operation is and how it would severely affect my quality of life. When you are faced with a choice of life-changing surgery or not surviving the cancer, it became an easy decision for my wife and I.

Before I could have the surgery, I had to undergo radiotherapy and chemotherapy, which was being done at a local NHS hospital. Thankfully my new boss was very understanding, and I went in five days a week to begin the radiotherapy.

After two weeks of radiotherapy, it was horrific. I had blocked bowels, diarrhoea, and constipation at the same time. I always was just a yard from the loo where I slept but many times I didn't make it. It was a terrible situation.

My kids were fourteen and eighteen at this point, which are quite vulnerable times and the first time we didn't tell them it was cancer as we had a solution to completely remove it. We told them post-surgery that I had cancer but it was now gone and not to worry

At this age you are pleased they are still childlike and focused on things that are no more than a foot in front of them, but at the same time, they have to comprehend it.

When it occurred again, it was still curative, and we told the kids what was going to happen, and they needed help to understand. I persevered with the radiotherapy and then the chemo and it seemed to do what we wanted.

I continued my Googling and tried to find the best surgeon to perform the surgery. There aren't many around, but I found one and my oncologist agreed with my research.

If I went ahead with the surgery, I would have had two external bags: one for poo and another for wee, and no prostate. It wasn't an ideal situation and back then if they had done the surgery, removed the cancer and my organs and told me I was free of cancer, I still would have taken it.

My new surgeon and I met after the handover from my oncologist, and he arranged another scan for me, to check before he scheduled the surgery. The scan showed six suspicious areas on my lung. I sat listening intently as he said, *"I'm not sure they look good, and we need to wait before I operate."*

He said he was concerned about carrying out this life-changing surgery if the cancer had spread to my lungs.

"The surgery is designed to take the cancer and quite a few of your vital organs out, and hopefully cure you, but if it has spread, why do a 12-hour mammoth operation which will completely alter your life, if we're looking at a life limiting or terminal diagnosis."

These were harsh words, and hope started to slip through the hour glass of my life.

After this meeting my new surgeon introduced me to his oncologist at a bowel cancer specialist hospital. They said systemic therapy was required, and they still told me it was curative.

I look back and I think how naïve I was. I wanted to be cured and I clung to this as my hope.

I did twelve rounds of chemo, receiving two types, as well as an immunotherapy treatment, which finished in November 2017, after which I had a scan in February the following year to check progress.

My wife and I were due to meet my oncologist on Monday 5th March 2018 to get my results.

There are some days that will always be burned into your mental DNA. Perhaps the day you got married, the days your kids are born and, without a doubt, the day you are told you have terminal cancer.

My wife and I went to get the results and we were the told the oncologist was ill. We were incredibly frustrated. Having prepared ourselves all weekend for this meeting, we felt very anxious at the time.

I said I wasn't accepting that we wouldn't get the results that day, as we had prepared ourselves for the results, and we wanted them. I said I wanted to speak to the radiologist that took my scan and they arranged for me to see him that day, at a separate hospital.

My wife and I drove to see him, and he was very accommodating, but it soon became clear that seeing cancer patients and explaining scan results wasn't his usual occupation. He had no bedside manner.

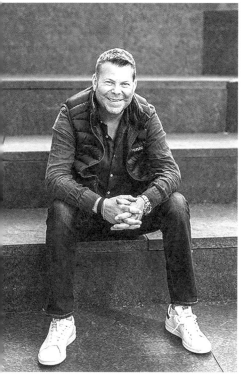

"I'm sorry to say that's it, you have to go home and get your affairs in order."

With one short sentence our lives had changed. It felt like a wrecking ball.

I was thinking, *"Oh my God, you just told me I'm going to die".*

Everything completely and utterly changed and even up to that moment, I had hoped I would be fixed. I couldn't believe what he just told us. We both went into shock.

The words tumbled out of my mouth as I asked, *"What are we talking?"*

"Years not months, but not many years."

"You mean two?"

The question hung in the air without an answer.

We had half an hour of him showing us my scans and I sat like a guppy fish, staring but not taking anything in. We were both on autopilot, staring but taking nothing in.

After our meeting we went to a restaurant, ordered the wine, and sat crying for a long time. Who knows what the staff thought, seeing us grip each other's hands and our wine glasses, with our faces wetter than the contents of the bottle.

One question kept coming back to both of us as we sat there staring at the ever-reducing wine.

What the hell do we say to the kids?

At that point there was no hope. Game over. This is the end.

Right there we made a pact not to tell the kids exactly what had happened until we'd gathered our thoughts. My oncologist called me the next day and tried to put a slightly different positive spin on the situation.

"Yes, its incurable, terminal in my opinion and you've probably got a couple of years."

My wife went into fix mode, and she found the Mulberry Centre, a charity at the Middlesex hospital, and they were outstanding. She arranged an appointment with a cancer trained nurse, and she really helped me. In one session she taught me coping mechanisms about time. *"Look at the clock, the hands are moving, time is passing, and you're still alive."*

That session was life saving for me. She lifted me off the ground and gave me hope. The first person to do so.

From that moment I started to build my own hope from the ground up and I knew I had to research my situation. My background in sales prepared me to set goals and targets and to figure out how to achieve them.

I found a local lady who had the same cancer as me, and she introduced me to a book; Radical Remission by Kelly Turner and that was my hope book. It gave me the confidence to figure things out and that led to finding Chris Woollam's book, Everything You Need To Know To Help Beat Cancer.

Through these books I had hope and faith in learning about my future journey.

Shortly after my diagnosis we went on holiday to Thailand with the kids and we told them the reality. We didn't sugar-coat it, and told them the truth which they understood.

When I knew I was on the way out, I started an Instagram page called the Bowel Bloke. I was aware of Deborah James, @bowelbabe. I called her to see if she was okay if I used that handle, and she was great.

I threw myself into fundraising and highlighting the symptoms of bowel cancer, and after a year of raising money for charity, I realised I couldn't keep milking my friends for money. I needed to get a wider public engagement.

I found it incredibly difficult to find men on forums who were willing to talk and having done some research, I found the vast majority of contributors on the forums were women, around 80%. The women I chatted to were amazing and so giving, but there were things I wanted to discuss where I needed a bloke who would understand the physical and mental issues that affect men.

I was looking for men dealing with an incurable cancer diagnosis, and if they had bowel cancer, it was a bonus.

The stats show that more men die of cancer, but there's no evidence that shows because we don't talk about it, we're more likely to die. Men are more isolated, we don't like sharing our feelings, and don't always find emotional support.

I thought, if I can't find what I want why not create it? I wanted to create an environment for men to get together, to provide information to help them, and offer a chance to support each other.

Sport seemed be a universal topic to get the conversation away from the medical aspects, and the idea for a cancer charity was born from meeting a cricket fanatic on one of the forums. Through my contacts I had arranged to take him to Lords, and I knew he wasn't well. Once I had it all arranged, I called to ask him if he wanted to come, and his wife told me he had died.

I still felt the idea had legs and with the help of some amazing people, I set up The Cancer Club, where men living with stage four cancer can share their interest in all types of sport. We look for companies and organisations that can arrange access to football, rugby, cricket, motor sport, or any other sports that members of the club want to take part in.

We managed to get it set up just before Covid, and suddenly there was no access to sporting events. This was a real blow, but we knew at some point we'd get back to some kind of normal, so we used this time to build our contacts and promote the club.

I hoped to help some people that had gone through a similar experience that I had, which might improve their life and give them the opportunity to find hope themselves.

We've arranged a few events and the feedback from the club members about the days out they've had together, with their family or friends, has been amazing. We had four seats at Wembley to watch football and I remember thinking *"if this day is the only one we manage, then we have achieved what I set out to do"*.

The nature of a club like this is that it's the sort of club you hope you'll never have to join, and you do lose members, but we hope we gave them and their family memories that will last.

I hoped to do something of value so that when I'm not here this club could live on and grow, and I'd love to create local groups in the UK, where people can go to events in their area.

I'm very proud of what we have achieved with The Cancer Club, and I still hope that I can be the 0.0001% that will survive. Failing that, I hope I can see out the important milestones, such as seeing my youngest child graduate and my eldest get his own house or get married.

I know I'm pushing the envelope as it's five years since my stage four incurable diagnosis, but I don't ever lose hope I can achieve these.

Matthew Wiltshire

It'll Be Fine

I'M GLAD I NEVER FELT A NEED TO COUNT how many times I said that in 2018. Every forlorn look, every hug, every moment of unknowing silence would always be followed by me telling anyone who would listen that, *"it'll be fine"*. God knows if I believed it or not.

Those words formed the mantra for what was easily the strangest year of my life to date. Most people remember the Beast from the East because it gave them some of their last snow days before the world's online infrastructure levelled-up overnight, forcing schools and offices to function virtually in the wake of the Covid pandemic. For me though, that storm in February 2018 holds memories of a wellied and frozen Kyle trudging sheepishly to the doctor's surgery to find out if the wee voice in his head telling him something wasn't quite right should actually be getting some airtime.

I'd noticed something maybe a week or two before and paid little to no attention to it. Why on that blizzard of a day I decided to jump over to get it checked, I guess I'll never know. It's fair to say now though that I'm pretty glad I did. The awkwardness of the situation couldn't be avoided—from my side at least—but I reckon getting the doc to check me out that day was probably worth the thirty seconds of numbing embarrassment.

I hadn't told a soul that I was going, so when I got given notice of my urgent ultrasound about three days later, I was almost annoyed that I had no-one to crack some incredible one-liners with about my upcoming ball scan. At this point I think some reality must have started to dawn, but I was still wholeheartedly ignoring the potentially tumour-shaped elephant in the room. I only know this because the day after my scan, I was due to fly to the States for work and I had done absolutely nothing to build any kind of contingency into my plans. I mean, what are the chances of me getting thrown a cancer diagnosis? Slim, no?

Apparently not slim enough.

The America trip didn't happen. It, along with life as I knew it, got shelved in one phone call. First came surgery, then it all kicked off. When we eventually found out that I had a non-seminoma teratoma—fancy name for testicular cancer—and that the cancer had hit my lymph nodes, none of us actually knew what it meant. We thought we knew but it was only when chemo and rounds were mentioned that we really sat up and took notice—yet again happily ignoring the low-key obvious until we really had to. I say *"we"* now because obviously I'd brought my parents into the fold by this point. My decision all along and, to this day one I've stuck to, was that I would go to all my appointments by myself. I don't really know why I want that, but it feels right that I get to tell them the news, and it also always meant that I had to make sure I understood everything before I relayed or abridged any info going their way.

I'd been standing outside the hospital after yet another scan when I took the decision that that moment was the right time to phone my mum and dump all of the ongoing chaos on her. The plan hadn't been to tell her while she was about to sit down for soup and a sandwich at a local garden centre, but that's what happened. I think it probably did ruin her lunch that day.

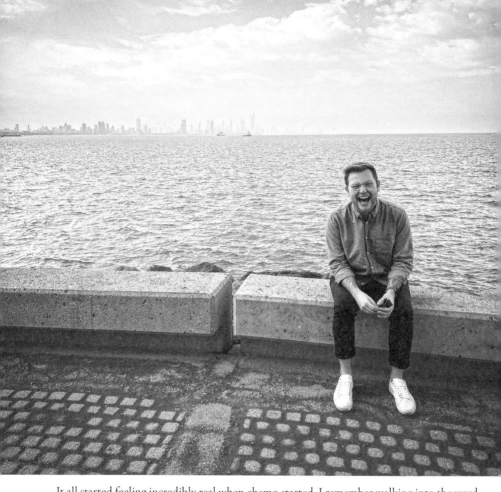

It all started feeling incredibly real when chemo started. I remember walking into the ward on day one for my first three-day in-patient chemo trip; no understanding or expectations, no knowing what 'chemo' was or actually meant, sick to my stomach with fear but a smile plastered across my face in hollow defiance of something much bigger than me.

Being a twenty-four, nearly twenty-five year old, I was fortunate enough to be treated on a Teenage Cancer Trust (TCT) ward. Being in my mid-twenties and very much not a teenager, this was as much of a surprise to me as it had to many of the young people before me. The sanctuary of this ward, the fact that it was filled with young people all unexpectedly traversing similar ridiculous mountains on their weaving strolls through life offered me an invaluable community to lean on, experts to listen to and friends who would ultimately offer the hope, as well as the humour, to keep me saying *"it'll be fine"*. The magic of this special collection of people was that it not only expanded my circle, but my parents and friends also found other parents and friends who they could ask questions of, learn things from, or more commonly, forget everything for a minute with.

All of this, of course, was foreign to me on that first day. The benefit of the TCT ward on day one was quite honestly the free wifi. I'd never been an in-patient before, but I had rocked up expecting analogue TV and the odd Sudoku, so the fact that scrolling Facebook and bingeing Desperate Housewives were options, was an added plus. After the initial infusion, a library of literature thrown in my direction, visits from allied health professionals and a weigh-in (that wasn't a highlight), I took the decision to post a photo to my Instagram. This was the first time that anyone outside my nearest and dearest was going to be told.

This move started what I've come to call the hurricane. Me at the middle of it, the eye of the storm, and everyone else: family, friends, neighbours, friends of neighbours, parents of friends, old teachers, pals' exes, the guy I pass on the way to work, people my granny knew in the 1970s, everyone creating some kind of weird storm around me. This storm is the way I describe cancer to anyone who asks. In the middle of it you move with the hurricane, silently trusting the process. Around you you're acutely aware of the emotions, the mechanics, the conversations but rarely, if ever, are they placed in front of you – everyone tries to make your life as easy as possible. Everyone puts on that brave face. Along with the metaphysical hurricane going on around me, for the rest of that day the vibrations and notifications on my phone more or less started a hurricane of their own. This was overwhelming. I never ever regret being open all the way through the weird times but that day my phone got thrown in a corner. I had mum to beat at Scrabble.

The small wins during chemo are not universal, but when they make an appearance, they make a difference. Sat in the ward the next day reading the messages of support I'd received was honestly heartwarming. It was the relationships that this ridiculousness had rekindled however, that became one of these rare wins. People I hadn't spoken to for years reached out and kick-started conversations years in the making. It shouldn't have taken a lump on my ball to make chatting to long-lost friends a reality, but it had, and I was over the moon.

As time went on going into the ward and getting set up with my machine beeping away next to me became almost normal. I had to have an injection every day, whether I was at the hospital or not, that also became normal. Blood tests every week, they became normal. My appetite peaking and troughing and anti-nausea pills becoming a necessity—all of this was normal too. When the time came, and despite my incessant effort to keep hold of it for as long as possible, unbelievably, having no hair also became the strangest of the normal. Before my hair thinned and I became scared of the rain in case it all went, the hair loss had been the thing keeping me up at night. It was going to be the bald arrow above my head everywhere I went saying that I was going through something. The day I decided to embrace it and got the clippers out, I didn't know whether to laugh or cry. To this day, I'm not actually sure which one won out. What I do remember is going out to meet my friends that night and realising en route that if wearing a cap meant saving on haircuts, at the same time as hopefully saving my life, then it would be fine.

Months passed and the normality of the weekly weigh-ins and the awkward parking situation outside the TCT unit just became everyday life. I'd made incredible friends, I'd got to spend more time with my parents, and thankfully, chemo hadn't hit me as hard as

I genuinely think it could have. Maybe I was lucky. One Saturday in September though I crossed the finish line. Treatment was over.

There's a strange thing about chemotherapy or, I guess, cancer treatment in general, where you just have to trust that it's doing the one thing it's supposed to do. The side effects tell you something's happening, and my bald head reminded me of that every day—but you never ever know what's actually going on. For me it was weeks, if not a month or two later, before I found myself back in the same room in the same hospital, with the same doctor, finding out if these bags of chemicals had actually done that one job they were supposed to do. Had it all been fine?

The fact that the scan showed that everything had gone, quite honestly didn't register. Despite knowing the incredible success rates of testicular cancer treatments, it wasn't success I'd focused on. I'd spent ages combing over the stats, arcanely and idiotically focusing in on the exceptions. I knew exactly what happened if that scan came back with no changes. I knew what surgeries we moved on to and where I'd have to go to have them carried out. It sounds silly now but for some reason, despite saying so regularly how fine it was all going to be, at that last moment, I gave in to the hopelessness of the situation.

Standing here now, on the other side of that weird year, I'm still in contact with the new friends and the old ones who reached out; my mum still can't seem to beat me at Scrabble, and I've never taken styling my hair for granted since. I think back to all those times I had no choice but to tell myself that everything would be okay, so that I could keep pushing forward. I realise now that they really are what got me through. I'm no expert by any means but as someone with a bit more experience than most, I really do wish I could promise that it will all be fine.

I can't do that but what I can say is that there's strength in hoping it will be.

Kyle Blain

Finding Hope in an Unexpected Place

I HAD BEEN HERE BEFORE. Eighteen months previously, I had an operation to remove stage two melanoma from my forearm and everything had gone to plan. The relief to be told the cancer hadn't spread was total, and, in the words of the person at the end of the phone, I could enjoy my weekend. It literally floored me. I still remember standing on that busy street in the heart of Edinburgh, breaking down and crying. Who knows what the passers-by thought of me, as I was crumpled with my back to the wall sobbing like a lost child, yet feeling the greatest relief.

Life carried on as normal and the scar on my arm was starting to heal quite nicely. It wasn't as angry looking as it had been and I had joked with my wife, Sophie, that I would have it turned into a snake tattoo, as it seemed to slither down my arm. She helpfully pointed out that I couldn't afford the divorce.

For eighteen months we lived, relaxed and took more joy from the simple things in life.

Then, in November 2019, I thought I had pulled a muscle in my back. The unplanned trip to A&E, due to the severe pain, had led to a very quick chain of events.

So here I was, back in the Western General Cancer Centre in Edinburgh, on my own. It was my choice to be on my own, which has to be the worst decision of my life. Fifty years on this planet and I still hadn't learned that you can't do everything on your own.

The large pale blue waiting room was filled with other people whose lives had been 'touched', or, more accurately, hammered by cancer. They sat patiently with a worried expression, which I would soon come to adopt, and along with their partners, friends and siblings, they sat waiting to see an oncologist.

What news would they get? Would there be tears, joy, despair, or even hope?

It didn't take long for my life to change. My softly spoken, incredibly polite oncologist started to talk and immediately I was enveloped in darkness. Not the kind of darkness where you can just switch on a light, or take off a cloak covering your head, but a fog of darkness, where the light of hope couldn't get in.

This was an out of body experience. Was he talking to me?

His words flowed over me, injecting me with a numbness and a freezing chill.

Stage Four, life limiting, incurable. These are the overall survival statistics, this is the treatment. It's quite a new treatment and if it works, we can hopefully extend your life.

Silence. I couldn't speak. I gathered the fragments of my thoughts and started to ask questions, but an hour later I would struggle to remember my questions, let alone the answers.

I called Sophie and asked her to come and meet me. I couldn't tell her over the phone and I needed her now, more than I ever could have known. Together we shared the despair, worry and grief of it all, and felt comfort and a lessening of the chill.

The main thought that ran through both our heads was, how do we tell the kids? There are no words anyone can find that describes the emotions experienced when telling your children that you have incurable, life limiting cancer. As young adults they took it incredibly well, but we could see the shock this left.

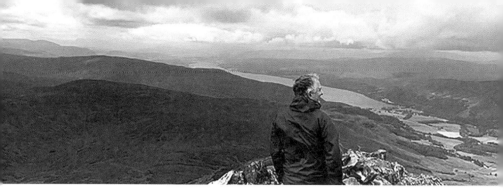

But there had to be hope. Where was it?

I told those close to me, family, friends, work colleagues, and I was determined this wouldn't define me. I wasn't cancer and cancer wasn't me.

I needed to find some sort of control and I wanted to share my cancer. Not everyone wanted to share, and it did feel selfish to thrust it upon them. It's hard telling someone and being met with complete silence. What do they say? What do I say?

I didn't expect people to take my cancer for me, but if we were to manage it, live with it, survive it, why should we do it alone?

I shared my cancer with my customers, along with my friend and colleague Marisa. Marisa knew the devastating impact that cancer had on her family and she soon became my new sister.

Marisa sat with me when I shared my cancer with my friends in that board room. Marisa didn't need to be there, but she wanted to be with me. Thank you, Marisa.

I shared my cancer with the people in that room, and to my complete surprise Kenny said;

"My brother in Australia has a company that tests the treatment you are going to receive. I'll put you in touch with him."

I couldn't quite grasp the enormity of what Kenny had said. His colleagues looked at him in complete surprise, as did Marissa and I. Could this be the hope we were looking for? Could Kenny's brother give me my missing piece to this cancer jigsaw?

We left that room in as much shock as our friends in there and I checked my phone every few hours, or even to be honest, every few minutes as my head was still spinning, for an email email from Kenny. He didn't disappoint and I quickly received his brother's email address.

I sent an email.

I got a reply.

I sat and read it with Sophie, and re-read it again and again.

Here was the hope we craved. Kenny's brother explained in simple language the power of the treatment I was to receive, the potential side effects and, more importantly, the chances of it working.

The suffocating fog has disappeared and our view of the world, and our future, was now looking more clear. We cried and smiled for the first time in days.

I shared my cancer, Kenny and his brother took it, and gave us hope in return.

Kevin Donaghy

Strong as a Tiger

I'VE ALWAYS BEEN A KEEN CURLER and, as skip of my team, it was my job to let the team know when to sweep and importantly, when to stop. I was known for my loud voice which would fill the rink and leave no one in any doubt what I needed them to do.

During one game in 2003, I wanted to let the team know what to do, but nothing came out. I thought it was strange. Then it happened a few other times. I didn't feel ill or notice anything visible in my neck, but this didn't feel normal, and it was affecting my game. I decided to see my GP about it.

I went to my doctor, and he sent me for tests and a tracheotomy, during which they confirmed that they had found a cancerous cyst and I would need an operation to remove it, then radiotherapy.

I'd like to think I'm a confident person and, working in HM Customs for most of my life, I've dealt with many tricky people and situations. There was nothing much that would faze me, until this.

It hit me very hard to hear it was cancer.

When I was told I had cancer I thought, how on earth has this happened? I've been very healthy. Walking and running were my thing and I'd done marathons and the Great North Run a few times, usually in a kilt and doing the odd Highland Fling for the spectators in the middle of the roundabouts!

So why me?

Is it my time to go?

I was 48 when I was diagnosed, and I thought, how do I address this?

I needed to get into some sort of pattern or plan on how to get through it.

Before my operation and I started my radiotherapy, I told my work I would go in early to the office, where I was the only member of staff, before I'd drive one hundred and twenty miles, there and back, to the hospital in Edinburgh for my treatment.

The cyst was removed without any complications, and I was more confident I could manage this but due to the pain from the radiotherapy and having to take drugs to combat that, I had to get someone to drive for me. I was determined the cancer wouldn't kill me, but the drive might.

My routine during the five-day-a-week radiotherapy sessions was to get up at 6am, drive the 15 miles to work, and then walk around the stunning Berwick-Upon-Tweed town walls (which had been built by King Edward I to keep the Scots out of England—but I still got in every day). I'd sit on the walls looking out at the North Sea and convince myself that the treatment would work. After this I'd do some work then go to Edinburgh, put on my mask, and be blasted.

It soon became obvious that my diet would be very limited and I survived on soup, porridge and custard—but not all in the same bowl. I would go to bed at 6pm, have my pain killers and try to sleep.

I felt organised and my routine helped me. During this time, I didn't want to see anyone other than my family, as I needed no distractions during my treatment, and it was hard to talk to people, which always felt awkward with long silences and pitying stares.

Nothing would interfere with my routine, and I'd concentrate so hard on getting better. I never doubted I would get better; I was quite adamant about that.

As I had convinced myself that the treatment would work, it was a relief to hear that it had, and with regular scans, which started at three months, then six, then yearly, I had been cured of cancer.

Fast forward a few years and in late 2021 I was going to the toilet a lot, especially in the mornings. I was walking with friends every morning for about an hour, and I was always needing to stop and wee. My friends would take the mickey out of me, and I knew at my age that this could happen, but I needed to know what was causing it.

I was referred to my local hospital for a consultation and tests and I saw the same consultant that had checked my prostate three years previously. His bedside manner wasn't the best, and I remember he said *"Don't contact me, I'll contact you"*, which left me feeling a bit chastised.

He had arranged a scan, following which he said whilst he didn't have all the information from it, it doesn't appear too serious.

Following my first scan, I was referred for another and following that scan I was advised over the phone, due to Covid restrictions, that it looked like prostate cancer, and they would need to operate.

I thought to myself, I've handled this once before so I will handle it again. I had no idea what this would involve, but I was determined to do it again.

I didn't know how serious and different to my first cancer this would be.

We discussed options with the consultant and he advised that I could opt for the surgery to remove all the cancer or radiotherapy to target it. He explained the impact that both might have on my future health and after talking this through with my family I opted for the surgery.

The hope was that this would be fully taken care of with the surgery and we could get on with our lives.

Due to Covid and pressures on NHS hospitals, I had to go to a private hospital in Edinburgh and I was advised I would spend one night in there and then I'd be able to go home. This sounded very hopeful and having beaten cancer before I went in with a positive mindset that I would do the same.

In the private hospital I wasn't feeling good after the surgery, where they had removed my prostate, the tumour, and a number of lymph nodes. I started to get sharp pains in my kidney as soon as I woke up. I was also very bloated, with my stomach swelling to the size my wife was when she was nine months pregnant! There was a lot of gas which wasn't coming out and this was very painful. The nurses were joking that they'd have to get the midwife in soon.

They decided they had to put stents into my kidneys. This could only happen at the NHS hospital in Edinburgh.

It was after midnight when I was transferred in a rickety old ambulance and the snow was coming down on my face as they tried to get the vehicle's doors closed, which took quite a while. It was an incredibly rough four-mile journey through Edinburgh and every pothole felt like a moon crater.

At the hospital I was put into a room and the nurses said they would have to insert a bile tube. I asked them if they had to do it at 2.30am, as I was feeling awful with the pain and just wanted to sleep. It was one of the worst experiences I had encountered. I felt I was in hell, and I couldn't find hope in any of this situation.

My lowest point was later that day when they said they would have to take me in and operate on my kidneys. I was in so much pain. The consultant said I would be in surgery within thirty minutes and as I was in so much pain, I asked the consultant if I was going to die that night? He reassured me I wouldn't.

My overriding hope was that the pain would be taken away. The staff were trying to distract me with some chat about football and at that point I had absolutely no interest in talking.

Thankfully the stents took pressure off my kidneys, and they could then get the fluid out of my body, though I still had a huge stomach. The nurses would call me *"beach ball"*. I took that with a smile and with the humour that it was meant.

I spent three weeks in the high dependency ward, which was a great place for me as I was looked after 24/7 by a fantastic team of nurses.

Once I left the hospital, I was told that incontinence would be a problem and I have struggled with this. I love the outdoors and have had to put a lot of my life on hold as I couldn't control my bowels. At the moment I can't go outside too much due to this incontinence. I use pads but if I have a few glasses of wine the taps are turned on. I went to a wedding the other month and had to go back to my room, I couldn't handle that every time I moved, I would leak.

I speak to a physio every month who shows a lot of empathy and advises me on exercises to help control this. She makes me understand I'm not the only person who experiences this, and this gives me hope. Thanks to her advice, pelvic floor exercises are now part of my routine, before and after the surgery, and I do them religiously three times a day. She reassures me it does get better.

I hope I can get more control so that I can spend more time outside, and I know it will get worse before it gets better. If you want the lovely view, you have to slog up the hill first.

When I went back to see my consultant after a few weeks, he said that they might not have got all the cancer. This hit me quite hard. They might have to give me some radiotherapy and hormone treatment.

I got quite down when I was told the cancer was still there. Some people may call it depression. I found it very hard to handle. I also had the stents in my kidneys for three months over summer and I couldn't walk or do anything without being in pain. I spent most of that time in bed.

I'm hoping if the cancer is still there that the treatment will knock it on the head and I can get back to some normality.

One of the biggest things that helped me with my mental challenges was a book The Magic in the Tin by Paul Ferris. It was recommended by a friend that had prostate cancer and he said it might help and it had some humour. It's a very emotional book where he describes his prostate cancer and I could resonate with everything he was saying. I could relate to his story, and he shared a number of things that the medical team don't always tell you.

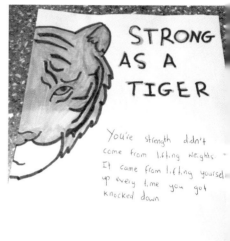

The book registered with me and I could feel what he went through, and he gave me hope.

Whilst I'm waiting for my treatment, I'll keep doing my exercises, and hopefully I can spend a bit more time walking.

We see our grandkids quite often. My eldest granddaughter is eleven and she sent me a card with a picture of a tiger on it and the words, *"Strong as a Tiger"* printed on the front. She wrote in the card, *"Your strength didn't come from lifting weights, it came from lifting yourself up every time you got knocked down."*

I read that card a lot and it's always very emotional when I do. It gives me immense hope, as does the amazing support I've had from my wife Judith and my daughters Gemma and Louise, without whom things may have been very different.

It's important to have goals in life and I use affirmations when I went through both my cancers and I keep telling myself I'm getting better every day, perhaps ten–twenty times a day. I'll make one up and use it for a while then move onto another one.

Thinking positively gives me hope.

Harry Brydon

A Bucketload of Hope

I WAS FIRST DIAGNOSED WITH BREAST CANCER IN NOVEMBER 2016, a few days after my thirty-ninth birthday.

I had found a lump in my right breast. I'd had a few lumps over the years and I would always get them checked out. The doctor would have a feel, tell me there was no family history, I was the wrong age and, thankfully, they were nothing sinister.

Following my previous visits, like a lot of people, I convinced myself it was nothing as I'm the wrong age and there's no family history, so it will be okay. It would be fine, and I put off doing anything.

It started to play on my mind so I mentioned it to my husband Mark that I had a lump and I wanted him to look at it. He was stood at the other side of the room, and as soon as I lifted my top, he said, *"Bloody hell, I can see it from here"*.

That worried and panicked me so I went to see my GP. He was brilliant. He had a feel and said he didn't know what it was, but he wanted to get it checked out.

He also asked if I felt anything under my arm and I said I hadn't, but I got the impression he might have. The GP didn't say anything at the time, but I should have known something was up. My mum was a Macmillan nurse, and this would have rung alarm bells.

I went to the cancer centre for a mammogram and took my husband and three-year-old daughter. My four-year-old daughter was at school. It never occurred to me that something could be wrong.

Just after the mammogram a nurse who had been in the room said *"good luck"*. This struck me as a very bizarre thing to say. Why would I need luck? Still, I thought, it won't be anything, I'm the wrong age, there's no history in the family, and I had breast fed both my daughters.

Straight after the mammogram, I went into an ultrasound with my husband and daughter. Halfway through, the atmosphere changed suddenly. The air turned to ice as the staff stopped talking and the radiographer leaned over and whispered, *"You need to ask your husband to take your daughter out of the room"*. They were sat behind the curtain and I started to panic. My immediate reaction was I wanted to just run out of the room and hospital and get as far away as possible, but I realised the problem was with me, not around me.

I opened the curtain and told my husband, as calmly as I could, that he needed to take our daughter out of the room. My husband asked why and probably saw the fear on my face, but I had nothing I could tell him at that point. I just asked him to take her out.

After they had left, the radiographer said she had seen something, and she would talk to me in a second. One of the nurses tried to distract me with small talk but I couldn't listen to her, my mind was racing.

I was told by the radiographer: *"I have seen something, we don't know what it is and we will have to do a biopsy, but it's not the end of the world."* It's not the end of the world. Out of the darkness came this tiny ray of hope. It's not the end of the world.

Okay, that's a good thing, isn't it, I asked myself?

So, it was out of radiology and into a biopsy there and then and by this time my husband and daughter were back in the room.

This is when I met an oncologist and I felt I was on a factory assembly line, getting passed from one department to another. The oncologist asked me what I'd been told and I just blurted out, *"It's not the end of the world,"* and everyone laughed.

The oncologist looked at me and said it probably is cancer, but we need to wait on the biopsy results.

Coming home I absolutely knew it was cancer. Call it mother's intuition, reading the room, picking up on what the nurse had said, or just a gut feeling; but I knew it was.

A week later, after the biopsy, they confirmed it was stage three invasive ductal carcinoma: breast cancer. I thought, this is it for me. There is no hope for me and my family. I must prepare myself and my family for life without me.

A few weeks later I had a single mastectomy and they removed sixteen lymph nodes under my arm. They found the cancer had spread to three of them.

Next stage was a full-body MRI and CT scan to check if the cancer had spread any further. I was petrified. My breast care nurse called to chat about something, I can't remember what she said, as all I wanted to know was what my scan results were. Scanxiety is real!

She confirmed it was good news. There was no further spread anywhere else in my body and she told me I would essentially be 'cured'. I wanted to run out the door screaming. I was so happy. It hadn't spread and suddenly hope was back, staring me right in the eye.

Since my primary diagnosis I had always thought I wouldn't live to be an old lady, but the thought of not seeing my two daughters grow up, get married and enjoy their lives had hung around me. Suddenly that was lifted.

There was hope now.

I wasn't done with the hospital though, and I had six rounds of adjuvant chemotherapy to stop the cancer spreading. I received two different types, one of which gave me the worst hangover I've ever had—which was saying something—and the other, the worst flu symptoms I'd ever had.

The same week that I was diagnosed with cancer, my husband had signed a lease to take on a new business venture. The lease was on a derelict post office, which he wanted to convert into a pub. It was always his dream to own his own business. Cancer is incredibly stressful, but we obviously needed a bit more stress. Talk about great timing.

Thankfully, my work were amazing and they gave me a year off on full pay. *"You need to take time off and get better, don't worry about working"*. This was massively appreciated and took a lot of stress away from us all, as my husband had given up his job.

At the same time as I started my chemotherapy, the work on the pub started and when I felt rubbish, I wanted to see how the pub was progressing. The project was due to finish at the same time as my chemotherapy treatment. It was strange, but I could track my progress which wasn't visible, by the progress we were making in the pub. When I saw the toilets going in or the walls getting painted, this gave me hope that my treatment would soon be ending.

One morning Mark said the lights were going up. I was feeling horrendous. I had no hair, one boob and I was feeling hungover and full of the flu. I needed to see this milestone achieved, and that gave me hope.

I was okay about losing my hair, but not my eyebrows or eyelashes. Eyebrows and eyelashes are the difference between rocking short hair and looking like a cancer victim.

We had amazing support from my mum and my husband's mum during my chemo. With my mum being a Macmillan nurse, she was with me during my chemo week, then my mother-in-law would come the following week when I felt a bit better, to help us get back on top of everything.

I have been so very lucky with my support network. Mark has been wonderful. Up until Covid, he came to every single hospital and doctor appointments with me. He has been right there at my side throughout this entire nightmare, despite having a new business to run, and two young children to look after. We talk regularly about our situation, and how we feel about it. I can lift him up if he's having a bad time, and vice versa. We are a proper team.

I've also had loads of practical and emotional support from my sister, who is only a year older than me and also has two girls the same age as my two. Plus there was help from friends and family, who have all rallied round to help us out with the girls, and to bring us meals without asking when we needed it most. My elder daughter had only just started school and it still amazes me now how the school mums, people I barely knew, could offer such support. Such simple gestures meant so much to us and made such a difference.

When I was first diagnosed, Mark's best friend came round with his wife, who's an oncology nurse. Mark's friend said something highly inappropriate given the circumstances, but very funny, and we all burst out laughing. It's weird how you can find humour in cancer, but sometimes it's better to laugh than cry.

I started a blog on my primary diagnosis so people could read and be updated, and they didn't have to call me up or pop round when I was feeling awful. It gave me something to do during chemo and as my memory was so terrible, I'd write it straight after. On reflection, I hope that my blog can help people going through the same experience.

After the chemo finished, I went back to work. The pub opened and when people asked if they could help us, we'd give them a mop and bucket and ask them to help us clean the pub. We were thankful to have had plenty of offers and often from the most unlikely places.

Life had returned to normal and I was told if I was two years clear of the treatment, following my primary diagnosis, then the chances of it coming back were massively reduced. Mark asked the oncologist, what if it comes back?

The oncologist said if it comes back in the breast we go through the same process. If it appears anywhere else, it's classed as secondary cancer and it's incurable.

As soon as we left the meeting I glared at Mark and asked him why on earth he asked that question? I've just left the gates of hell and the last thing I wanted to think about was re-entering them again.

On hindsight it was a good job he did ask.

I was coming up to my two-year post treatment anniversary and I started to get a pain in my hip. I was on a medical trial and at the end of one of the meetings I mentioned the pain which I put down to a running injury.

They said they would arrange the scan to check and I asked if it could be cancer again. I was reassured it probably was a running injury, but the scan would confirm this.

I didn't know secondary cancer could come back in your bones, but the nurses did. They said if it's nothing we'll tell you over the phone, but if it is something we'll ask you to come in.

I had the scan and I carried on not thinking too much of it and I then got a phone call at work from one of the nurses I'd spoken to.

"Hi Kathryn. It's Gill from The Christie, we've got your scan results. Can you come in tomorrow?"

NO NO NO NO NO NO NO!

I was like a wild animal pacing up and down, and who knows what my heart rate was, but it was going off the scale.

"This is bad isn't it? Is it bad?"

"I can't tell you over the phone."

"Well, you can't not tell me now." I probably screamed this.

I was asked to get someone with me and after I'd physically grabbed a startled colleague, I asked her if my cancer was back, and she said yes.

Something immediately clicked and I flipped from panic into action mode and said I'd be there tomorrow at 1pm. I changed from a scared, caged animal into survival mode.

I had to call Mark and I asked him if he was with our kids. He said he was, and I said move away from them right now, which I know scared him, and then I told him it was back.

This was twenty-three months after finishing my primary treatment and I was so close to hitting the two-year mark.

The next day I met my oncologist again, who was the loveliest man, which certainly helped. He asked if I wanted to know timescales and I said, *"Yes, no, yes, no, I do if it's good but not if it's bad. But then if you don't tell me I'll know it's bad. "*

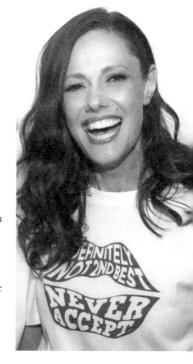

I was still having this terrible debate with myself, when he said, *"We're talking years, not months.".*

It's still not long enough, but I had convinced myself that I wouldn't see that Christmas. After taking all my hope, I now had a bit back. If I focus on each day at a time this would help us.

One of the best pieces of advice I was given upon my terminal diagnosis was don't make any drastic decisions in the first six months. Our minds had immediately raced to giving up work, selling the pub, selling the house, getting a dog. We weren't thinking straight, as no one probably does when you receive this kind of news. We took the advice and didn't make any immediate changes.

I needed to keep busy after this diagnosis and I didn't want to stay at home dwelling on my hopeless situation. I only cried once after my primary diagnosis, whilst accidentally sitting on my phone and bum-calling my best friend who could hear me crying, I heard them shouting *"what's going on?"* and I immediately stopped crying and started laughing. We still laugh about it.

My daughters were so young and I didn't want them to know, so we had a no cry policy and knew we had to be strong for them.

We had told the kids that *"mummy was poorly"* during my primary diagnosis and that my hair would fall out as the medicine is so strong, which made them both giggle. I was determined I wouldn't spend days in bed. I remember dragging myself out, even on the worst days, so they wouldn't see me in bed being ill. I still did the school runs most days, but some days I only made it to the sofa.

I'm a teacher and had researched how to talk to children about a cancer diagnosis, so felt equipped to talk to my girls and explain what was now happening. We told them the cancer had come back and was now in my bones. We explained that there was no cure and that I would have to take medicine for the rest of my life, but this time the medicine wouldn't make my hair fall out.

They've grown up with mummy having cancer and the saddest part is they will only ever remember the cancer version of me—not what I was like before. Mark does everything around the house now as I'm always so tired outside of work, and the other day they said daddy always makes our tea, you don't mummy. I reminded them I used to always make their tea when they were little, from breast-feeding them both for the first year of their life, to steaming and blitzing vegetables daily, but they've forgotten.

I met up with a school-mum-friend one day shortly after my secondary diagnosis. She had lost her mum suddenly when she was just six years old. She talked about her experiences and gave me loads of sound advice. It was from that conversation that I decided to embark on reading Harry Potter to Ruby and Nancy. I would read the book to them every night, then as we finished each one, we would watch the film (with Mark, so he could join in our discussion on it around the dinner table most evenings!). I am now coming up to four years of reading Harry Potter to my girls! We are on book number six, so getting there! My hope is that it gives my girls something tangible to hold on to: them knowing that I have read every single one of the words in those books, and that they will always have that even when I'm no longer here.

Following the diagnosis, I was put on medication which was part of the trial I was on, but I was in the control group, so it was time to start the real thing.

I was medically pushed through the menopause so that I could start the cancer treatment, Palbociclib, which targets your hormones as my type of cancer feeds off them, therefore limiting its progress. It was horrendous being pushed through an early menopause. It felt like a form of torture, for all of us.

I had started my cancer treatment just before the first Covid pandemic, and I was told that I had to immediately stop taking the drug as they compromised my immune system and they were worried about me catching Covid, as they didn't know what would happen if I did.

At this point the biggest risk to my life was Covid rather than cancer. We had decided to isolate just before the first lockdown was announced so I stopped work, the kids came out of school, and we closed the pub.

For fourteen months we locked down and didn't see anyone, apart from through the window or sometimes we'd take our caravan and park it in our parents' drive and chat through the closed window.

Like most people we thought this would only be for twelve weeks. Luckily our daughters were young enough to want to be at home with the family and old enough to be a bit more independent, so we didn't have to constantly watch them.

How could we cope with twelve weeks of not leaving the house, let alone fourteen months? My sister changed my thought process. She said you have time with just your family and following everything you've been through you now get time that you wouldn't have had. You need to see this as a positive. From that moment we did and, as a teacher, getting to teach my own kids for over a year was a perfect scenario.

I had to have Zoladex injections every month to keep me in a state of menopause, and I was petrified to go to the GP surgery to get these, as I might pick something up. It had to be administered by a health care professional and luckily my dad was a GP. I contacted my GP and asked if my dad would be able to administer this. Thankfully it was approved, and my wonderful dad would drive fifty miles, don full PPE, then we would meet in my driveway, he would inject me, then drive home.

My cancer was in my spine and pelvis and after stopping the treatment for three months, due to Covid, it had now moved to my liver.

As the first Covid wave subsided it was decided that I should come off Palbociclib and move onto an oral chemotherapy treatment of Capecitabine. This was two years ago and thankfully the cancer has disappeared from my liver and it's just in my spine and pelvis. This new drug is so manageable, I'm out of the menopause and the only real side effects are on the palms of my hands and soles of my feet. They're itchy and raw looking. Mark went to hold my hand the other day and recoiled saying, *"your hands feel like feet"*, which really made me laugh. I'm really conscious of this if I have to shake hands with anyone.

Today I've got hope in bucketloads. I don't dwell on my situation, though it is always there.

I don't have 'The Fear' that I first had with my primary diagnosis. There is hope that I might see my daughters go to high school, and maybe even get to meet their first boyfriends. And who knows… I may even see them get married! I never really had an option of giving up with my girls being so young. Everything I did was for them.

I know some women live with secondary breast cancer for years and I hope that's going to be me. I'm fit, I feel healthy and if I just keep running towards life, I feel like it won't catch up with me.

My girls know I have cancer, but they've never asked what it means ultimately. We are always honest and open with them, normalising our situation. I've never volunteered that it's terminal. I think that if they haven't asked then they're not ready to hear the answer. I'm part of a group of twenty women that got together for a photo shoot to raise awareness of secondary breast cancer and it's a photo I'm so proud of. We had hoodies made recently, which have the slogan *"fighting to be heard"* on the front and the names of five women who have since left us on the back. When I first wore my hoodie, my ten-year-old daughter asked me what the names were on the back of the jumper?

I said, *"They are the ladies from the photo that have sadly died."*

"They've died?" she asked.

"Yes," I said.

I could see her taking this in and then she said, *"Okay"*.

They don't know the treatments will run out at some point but there's always the hope that there are new ones round the corner, so we will broach that subject as and when we need to in the future. There is a fine line between being honest and ruining their childhood.

I am now living my life to the full: still working full time as a teacher, but living in the moment and having a great time. I am generally a positive person and, at the time I was diagnosed, I would have loved to have known somebody with secondary breast cancer that is living a normal life. This is what I'm determined to do.

One of my main aims has been to help other people in my situation. Since my breast cancer diagnosis, a few people within my circle of family and friends have also been diagnosed with breast cancer, including my lovely sister-in-law. A cancer diagnosis can make you feel very lonely, even when you're surrounded by people. I was glad I was able to support them and offer advice. I have managed to build up a social media presence and am regularly approached by strangers who are going through a primary or secondary breast cancer diagnosis themselves or are supporting someone close to them who are going through it. I am (relatively) young, a mum, a wife, and a teacher who is trying and succeeding to live as normal a life as possible. I haven't given up, I haven't crumbled and I don't dwell on my future. I live in the moment and still see so many positives in life. I want to help other cancer patients to do the same.

My aim is to spread hope as far and wide as I can... as there is life after a terminal diagnosis.

Kate Rackham

Charity Begins at Home

I **TRY TO GIVE HOPE TO PEOPLE.** Setting up a cancer charity was something I had never planned to do. I saw myself as continuing my career in law, bringing up my kids and looking after my dogs, then my husband (that's the order in my house!)

Our family had been long-suffering Oldham Athletic fans which led me to tinker with online forums in the early 2000s. I saw a post from a young lad named Jon from Larne in Northern Ireland, asking if anyone knew anything about Barrow-In-Furness.

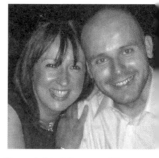

I replied, quite cheekily and not too flatteringly about the town, and Jon told me that he was getting his first job out of university working there. Jon wasn't an Oldham fan, he supported Glasgow Rangers, but we soon made a connection as I had family living in Barrow.

We met up with Jon when he started his new job, and he quickly became a very dear friend and part of our family. We hadn't known Jon that long when his journey with cancer started. Looking back now, that period of six years where we supported Jon and his family as his melanoma spread and eventually took his life, seems like such a short period of time in which we loved and lost too quickly.

Throughout this time, I became a Google expert on melanoma cancer and I soon realised there were no options to cure the cancer or keep it at bay for any length of time. Chemotherapy and radiotherapy were able to prolong life, but they were quite ineffective at stopping its progress.

Jon died one month after he turned thirty, and I decided that this wasn't right, that a young man had no options, and hope had been taken from him, his family, and his friends.

Following Jon's death, I had a burning desire to do more and help more people. It seemed crazy that there were no effective treatments for melanoma, and in my spare time I dedicated myself to being involved in the search for hope.

This is how Melanoma UK was born and, whilst juggling family life and work, my family and I got involved. We had supported Jon during his regular trips to The Christie cancer centre in Manchester and this seemed an obvious place to start.

A few months before Jon passed away, I spoke to his oncologist and asked how we could help other people living with melanoma. I was told that £250,000 was needed for a particular piece of research. I had told Jon that I was going to start doing something to support people like him and the teams who were treating melanoma patients. After all, those medics needed to be able to offer hope to patients, didn't they? Imagine being a doctor and never being able to offer any hope to your patients?

So we started fund raising and we grew our contacts in research and government, and soon became a vital part of the melanoma community.

Whilst doing this I was still working full-time and being a mother, daughter and friend.

One of my colleagues asked me why I was not dedicating all my time to Melanoma UK. And suddenly, it made sense. I was meant to be doing this.

I'd created something that I couldn't walk away from. Indeed, I didn't want to. My colleague helped me to set it up formally as a charity and that gave me the push I needed to focus full-time on this work.

I walked into my senior partner's office with my envelope, and he knew what the white envelope meant. He asked me if I was joining another firm, and I explained that I was now going to dedicate my time to Melanoma UK. His response was that he and the partners knew I would do this at some point, so I left with their blessing.

In formally setting up the charity I wanted to carry on from where I thought we had left off and give more time and support to the patients. We were being contacted by more patients and families and it was clear that helping The Christie to fundraise was the start and not the end.

When Jon was going through his cancer treatment, he would often say that he wished there was another melanoma patient he could speak to. During his treatment, he had not come across anyone with melanoma and this left him feeling terribly isolated.

I wanted to get melanoma patients together to share experiences, their stories and more importantly their hope. I just wanted to put my arms around the patients and help in any way I could.

If you'd asked me about hope in 2006, it wasn't a word that meant too much to me or melanoma patients, as the current treatments we have now didn't exist then.

I hoped Jon would survive melanoma, and he didn't.

I hoped doctors would find a miracle cure for him, and they didn't.

Your best hope was that a patient would have a peaceful and pain free end of life.

There wasn't a lot of hope in our world then.

There have been many times when I felt without hope. We were involved in our first UK Melanoma drug appraisal with NICE back in 2011, which was an alien experience for me. Hearing that the drug was not approved for patient use left me feeling completely hopeless. For once, in the history of melanoma treatment, we had the opportunity to help get a life-saving drug approved. Yet the decision had gone against us. I felt as is we had let people down, people who were constantly searching for hope.

With the bad news, I was personally devastated, and I felt like I had wasted my time and given false hope. How could I tell our patients that this had been refused? It felt like all hope had gone.

Having slept on the disappointment, the next day I had renewed hope and I looked at this as a temporary setback. Working with patients and MPs who I had got to know, we created a dossier that would support the appeal. The purpose was to demonstrate why patients needed this treatment.

Six months later, after a re-submission, the drug was approved, and we had the first life extending treatment for melanoma in the UK.

This might seem like a short period in time, but in the life of a melanoma patient, this was the average life expectancy after a stage four diagnosis.

I've never experienced melanoma and I don't know what goes through our patients' heads when they lay down at night, though I have held the hands of a lot of patients and seen them in various stages of the disease. Many will cling to hope as they feel there is nothing else.

A patient once said to me all he had was hope and without it, he would be lost.

We're very hands-on, at the coalface, and I think we've made a difference to patients. We are always at the end of the phone for them and their family members. I know we fill a gap in their needs, outside of the medical support they get.

We now have a bank of patients that have situational experience, and we ask them to talk to new patients that have been recently diagnosed. We must take care in matching them to ensure that they have shared experiences and whilst it's incredibly scary, talking to someone who is living with cancer can be invaluable.

We have a small army of great listeners and givers of hope, and this is something we are very proud of, as sometimes only those that have walked that path will know how to guide.

Whilst treatment for melanoma has advanced in the past ten years with the innovation of immunotherapy, we don't have a cure and it still takes too many lives.

For those approaching end of life, it's hard to give hope. In my experience the patient and their family aren't looking for hope. All we can do is listen and use our experience and training in bereavement counselling to support them in their need to know what comes next.

People think that grief comes after death, but in my experience, it can come earlier: a living grief, which can be hard to understand. We are there to listen and there are times when that is all that's required. Someone to listen.

What does hope mean now?

I look back on the fifteen years I've been involved with skin cancer, and I hope we are helping our community. That is where my hope comes from. The stories of success grow every year and that continues to give me hope.

I hope that as the years progress and when I eventually hand the reins over, we have created more awareness of melanoma and non-melanoma skin cancers and that science progresses to the point where we have a cure.

Hope and hoping means so much more than it did when Jon was first diagnosed.

Where there's hope, there's life. If you're not hoping, you're not living.

Gill Nuttall, Melanoma UK CEO

Jon's story
https://www.melanomauk.org.uk/meet-jon-the-reason-we-are-here

Maggie May Help

WE NEVER THINK THAT WE WILL GET CANCER and, although over the years we know friends, family and colleagues that have cancer, it never crosses your mind that you will get it, until you do.

I have now had three different types of cancer. Each had varying degrees of seriousness and the impact it can have on your mental health is something you're not always made aware of.

Fifteen years ago, a good friend of mine was diagnosed with testicular cancer and after chatting to him and learning how he discovered it, I decided to check myself and I found something unusual.

I arranged a physical examination and an ultrasound via my GP, and it was very quickly determined that I probably had it too. There was no biopsy or further tests, I was told there and then that it was cancer, and I would need an operation soon.

There's not much that can prepare you for a cancer diagnosis, and I certainly wasn't prepared for it, the first time.

In a very short space of time, I had an operation and within a few weeks they had tested it and confirmed it was cancerous. With this type of cancer, if it's left unchecked it can move to your chest and brain, and if I hadn't spoken to my friend, this might have happened to me.

I was quite fortunate that I only had one dose of chemotherapy. At this time John Hartson, the Celtic footballer, had to have a brain operation as his testicular cancer had spread and he admitted it was partly due to not getting checked early enough.

There wasn't a lot of time between my initial check, diagnosis, operation and chemotherapy and whilst I'm quite a laid-back person, working in a high-pressure workplace, during this time I experienced an incredible bout of anxiety, and this scared me more than the cancer.

Just after my initial diagnosis I felt sheer panic. I couldn't sleep at night, and I didn't know what was going on. I found it incredibly hard to concentrate at work and I wanted to hide my feelings from my wife and young kids, as I felt I had to be strong for them.

Keeping anxiety to myself didn't help me or my family and it was only when I confided in my friend who had gone through the same cancer and procedures, that he told me he had felt the same way. He explained it's quite a normal reaction to a cancer diagnosis and the relief I felt after speaking to him was enormous. I wasn't alone, and he had given me hope by sharing his story.

I was also reassured by my oncologist that there was a very positive outcome expected, with three-monthly scans to check it hadn't spread, but I shouldn't take anything for granted. I didn't.

During this period, I hardly took any time off work and when our HR director asked me why I came back to work so quickly, I explained that by working and behaving normally, I hoped it would take my mind of it. It didn't, and I was probably far less effective at work than I thought I'd be.

Life returned to normal and with healthy scans every three and six months, I began a new venture with a friend of mine and we started our own company. I was incredibly busy and very happy.

In July 2019 I was in my car when I caught a glimpse of my throat in the rear-view mirror. I saw a lump and thought it looked quite strange and out of place. I went to see my GP to get it checked out and he thought it was unusual and asked if I'd had mumps as a kid. I said I had.

He referred me to the local Ear, Nose and Throat (ENT) clinic and said it was probably a branchial cyst, which forms when you're in the womb and can present at any time in your life and wasn't too serious.

The ENT consultant put a syringe in my neck and took out the fluid, reducing the lump to a small patch on my neck, and a few days later they confirmed that the tests were inconclusive.

Two weeks later the lump was back, and as I was going on holiday the next day I wanted to do something about it before I went. That evening I went to see a friend who's a GP and he removed the fluid and said the colour is consistent with it not being cancerous. So I went on holiday and we all had a great time. It never occurred to me that this was anything serious.

When I came back from holiday, I went back to ENT and had the lump removed and again the tests were inconclusive, but this time they also decided to remove one of my tonsils.

Following this procedure I went to see my consultant, who was an amazing lady, and just before my wife and I went into her office, she pulled the Macmillan nurse into the room. I knew at this point it wasn't going to be good news.

She said it was cancer but thankfully it was a tiny cancer. She explained she had only removed one tonsil as having both of them removed was very uncomfortable in later life and at this point she didn't think it was necessary.

I had cancer. Again.

Removing cancer from your neck or throat can be very complicated due to the nerves in your neck, and the consultant confirmed my cancer was based on the HPV virus, which in females presents in the cervix and for men it can appear in the throat.

I was unlucky having cancer twice but I felt lucky in that I had two cancers that, when caught early, could be treated and managed. Her confidence that this could be successfully treated gave me hope.

My consultant explained that it's a very well-trodden path and that I would have thirty sessions of radiotherapy, five days a week for six weeks. I'd also get two doses of chemo mid-way through and there was an additional eight per cent better outcome if I had the chemo.

She also explained that I would have a feeding tube for six weeks during the radiotherapy. I was quite stubborn and I refused the feeding tube. I didn't want to be fed through my nose and felt that I could manage the treatment without this. She explained only five–ten per cent of patients can get through the treatment without the tube.

I came to regret my decision.

I felt sick at being told my diagnosis and I wondered if my anxiety would return. Even though I was half prepared for the diagnosis, the thought of going through this treatment was a body blow. I had beaten cancer once, my business was doing very well, and here I was back having to deal with the disease.

I wanted to know the potential outcomes and gather as much information as possible whilst we were in her office. She said that whilst they can't guarantee any outcomes, based on the results and the fact that it's HPV-based, they would be treating me to try and cure me, rather than managing the cancer. This absolutely gave me hope.

My wife and I went to the pub straight afterwards, as it seemed like the best thing to do.

In preparation for the radiotherapy I was fitted for a head brace, which is a kind of papier-mâché mask. I would be bolted to the table so I wouldn't move and the radiotherapy could target the right area. I felt like Hannibal Lecter and every Monday to Friday for six weeks I put my mask on and was blasted with radiotherapy.

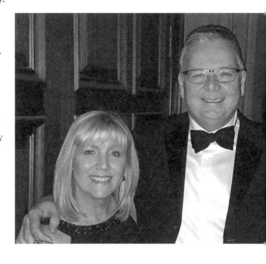

I tried to have as positive an outlook as I could, but the gruelling treatment took that away. I don't think I thought about hope then. My overriding hope was for the radiotherapy to end and to be told I was okay.

I soon began to unravel at the brutality of the treatment and, whilst the weekends were a great relief when I wasn't having treatment, my anxiety returned with a real vengeance and I started to lose weight.

I found that walking was the only way I could reduce my anxiety and I'd take my wife out walking in the rain and wind, at any time of day. I'd sleep, wake up, go for a walk, then go back to sleep again.

I was trying to function at work and at this point I was running my own business with my business partner. I was trying to remain positive, but I was non-functional. My business partner said I should take my mind off the treatment with work, but this wasn't the answer. I'd be in meetings and I'd have to leave the room as I could feel the anxiety coming on and I knew I couldn't concentrate. I needed to leave and I needed the people that came to my home to see me, to leave me alone.

The anxiety would well up and suddenly—bang—it consumed me.

My anxiety was all-consuming and I knew it was taking a toll on my family. I confided in the staff at the hospital, and I was advised to go to the Maggie's cancer centre with my wife.

The staff at Maggie's were amazing and confirmed it's one hundred per cent normal to suffer from anxiety, and it's my body's flight or fight response. I felt as if Maggie's were waiting for me and my second diagnosis.

I threw myself into the activities that they offered, and my family would accompany me to Tai Chi, reflexology, meditation and anything else I tried.

I was also walking lots in any spare time I had and I remember going to a keep fit class at Maggie's one afternoon. The instructor asked me to talk about any exercise I'd done the previous day. I said I'd done thirty-thousand steps on four walks that day and she nearly fell over. We had a good laugh about it.

Maggie's and walking helped to manage my anxiety but my lack of weight became an issue. On Christmas Eve at 4am I woke my wife and said I didn't feel good. I called the cancer centre and was admitted within an hour. Afterwards my family told me they were very worried I wouldn't come out. Within a few minutes of being admitted I had a feeding tube inserted and my physical recovery started.

It wasn't long after this that my treatment ended, and my physical and mental recovery continued. I saw a Macmillan counsellor, post-treatment, where we would talk about the physical and mental impact of the treatment and I amazed myself that after only two sessions I called them and said I feel so much better, and I never went back.

Life went back to normal, apart from Covid, and I threw myself into my business which is doing well. Thinking I had had enough cancer to last me the rest of my life, I recently had cancer removed from the bottom of my eyelid, and I've been told not to worry as it's been removed and there is no treatment that I need. Strangely my anxiety didn't return and perhaps this is a good sign.

Looking back, Maggie's played such an important role for my family and myself. They were the providers of my hope and they saved me. They are now the official charity for our business, and I'd recommend anyone who is diagnosed with cancer to have a chat with them.

I do hope that cancer is finished with me, as I'm certainly finished with cancer.

Alan Turnbull

Melanoma is a Bugger—or at least it can be

MY STORY PROBABLY STARTED MANY YEARS AGO when I was seven and my parents moved to Spain. They both loved sitting out in the sun and soaking up the rays. This was long before British people fully understood the long-term damage the sun can do. We didn't have suntan lotion, let alone high-factor sun screen. Mum even used olive oil to bake in the sun. Which is why we were probably not as careful as we should have been, and I got sunburnt a few times. I have fair hair, freckles and skin that was designed for rainy mountain tops rather than scorching sun. It only takes a few minutes in the midday sun for me to go from fair to pink to red and the sun even manages to find its way into my scalp. Peeling was a standard part of a Spanish summer.

And that's almost certainly when the damage was done.

Spool forward to Christmas 2018. I had just had my hair cut rather short for Christmas and the family was gathered in the kitchen in our house in Porth. My husband Jared was standing behind me and asked, *"What's that on the back of your head?"* I had felt something there for a while, but I get an itchy scalp and I thought it must just be a spot.

When Jared showed me a photo of the back of my head, I could see a raised mole. It was the size of a thumb nail, varying in colour from ruby to pink and yellow, and an odd shape. If I saw one of those today I would know exactly what I was dealing with, but back then I was more interested in getting the turkey in the oven and I dismissed any worries I might have had.

Three weeks later it was my birthday—11th January—and I was driving past my doctor's surgery. For some reason the mole came back into my head, and I decided to pop in to get it checked out. I was very lucky. Someone had just cancelled an appointment and they saw me a couple of hours later. The doctor didn't sound worried. He thought it might be a wart, but just to be careful, he was going to send me to the dermatologist as an urgent case.

Ten days later I was at the Royal Glamorgan Hospital. The dermatologist didn't sound all that worried either but she did think it was worth taking it out—and she made an appointment there and then for me to come in the next week.

That round of surgery was pretty simple. I was awake throughout and all I could sense was the doctor shaving a bit of my head before cutting out the mole and then pulling on the skin to close up the wound. The nurses were hilarious – dancing to Abba and Kylie through most of it. And I joked that at least I was getting a bit of a face lift in the process as they tautened the skin on my head. There was just one dark moment. I asked the doctor what she thought. *"Well, it's quite thick..."* she said.

Then it was a question of waiting. At first I was told it might be five weeks before I would hear anything but when I mentioned this to a doctor friend who is an MP, she said it shouldn't take anything like that long and I should push to get my results as soon as possible.

Then the receptionist called. They had the results, and could I come in two days later? They suggested that I might want to bring someone with me.

So, Jared and I sat in the waiting room at the Royal Glamorgan on a Thursday morning. I don't think either of us was really worried. He thought it was just routine. And I only had the slightest worry, presuming that if it was cancerous, it would be a stage one or two at the most. Inevitably I interpreted everything about the appointment. I persuaded myself it must be good news because I was booked in at 12.50, presumably therefore only allowing ten minutes.

In fact, it was about 1.30 before we were called in. My heart sank when I saw the doctor was sitting behind a desk, with a folder in front of her, looking very serious. That didn't augur well.

She got straight on with it. *"I have to tell you that it was quite a thick melanoma, and it had a little satellite, meaning that we would call it a stage three B melanoma."*

"How many stages are there?" I asked.

"Four," she said.

"And what are my chances?"

"Of living?"

"Of dying?"

"Well it's never precise and there are lots of things to take into consideration, but roughly forty percent chance of living a year."

Gulp. I held the table in one hand and Jared's hand in the other and I cried. She then explained what would happen next.

The next month involved an appointment with the maxillofacial surgeon who explained the next round of surgery and shared the fact that ground-breaking new targeted and immunotherapy drugs had been licensed by NICE for stage 3 melanoma only two weeks before I had turned up at the doctor. It would mean monthly appointments with an oncologist, which might be easier in London if I wanted to continue working in Parliament during my treatment.

The second round of surgery at the Prince Charles Hospital in Merthyr Tydfil involved carving out a much bigger chunk of skin off the back of my head and filling the hole with a graft from my tummy. As I was lying on the trolley waiting to go into surgery, one of the doctors popped in to thank me for my work as an MP.

This time I was under a general anaesthetic, because they would have to turn me over and apparently, I was very funny when I came round. Oddly enough, it was the day that several MPs left the Labour Party and set up on their own. I knew it was coming – they were all close friends – so I tweeted before the anaesthetist put me under that I would never leave the party, just in case anyone thought that my silence meant that I was also leaving.

The next day I was back in work in Parliament. The operation left me looking a bit like Frankenstein's monster, stitched and stapled together, so I had no choice but to talk openly about what I was going through. I decided that it might also encourage other people to get their suspicious moles checked out, so I did a round of interviews – and got cross when Kay Burley got me to cry on her show.

I still felt terrified that I was going to die but then I met my oncologist, Dr Mark Harries at Guy's Hospital, who explained the new treatments. I could either have an immunotherapy

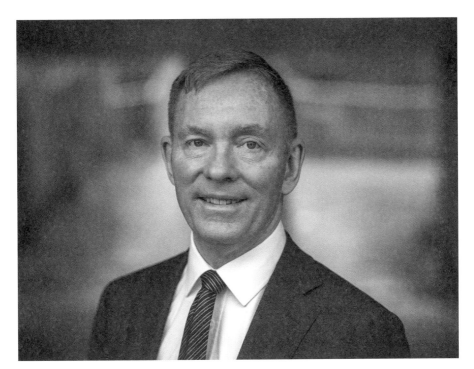

infusion every three weeks or, if my melanoma was BRAF positive, I could have targeted therapy in the form of five pills a day for a year. There might be side effects, but the evidence showed that either therapy would improve my life chances from forty per cent to ninety or even ninety-five. In addition, they would regularly pass me through an MRI and PET CT scanner to check that the melanoma hadn't spread anywhere else.

Amazingly, I had no side effects and I had just finished the course when Covid hit, so although I was initially told to shield, they soon decided I was at no greater risk than anyone else. Now I get checked or scanned every three months—and that will continue for another two years. Then it's every six months.

It's taught me a lot: the importance of a free healthcare system, the value of checking things out and the amazing advances in medicine. And I feel fortunate that the new drugs had just been licensed, that I had a husband who could spot it, that my husband did spot it when he did, that I didn't go into denial about it, and that the doctors and nurses were so utterly professional. They don't quite give you the all-clear with melanoma for ten years, and I thank the people who set up the NHS and work in it with all my heart, because I think I'll be around for a good while yet.

Chris Bryant, MP

Photograph by Phil Warren

The Glass is Always Half Full

2017 WAS TO BE A LANDMARK YEAR. I hit sixty years old in January and kicked off the year with a large party for family and friends. It was also the year my eldest son turned thirty, so a couple of sixty and thirty father and son celebration trips were planned. The first of these was a trip to Islay for the Fèis Ìle, the annual whisky festival in May, as we are both lovers of a single malt.

While on this wonderful—and somewhat intoxicating trip—I noticed a slight bump on the side of my neck while shaving but, as I had been suffering from a cold the week before, I just assumed it was my glands that were slightly swollen so didn't think much about it. When it was still there a week or so later, I booked to see my GP, who took a look and said if it was still there in two weeks, come back in. It wasn't causing any issues, so unfortunately, like most blokes I suppose, I didn't think to go back to see my GP until about six weeks later.

On this second visit I was examined again and given a letter for an urgent cancer referral, but to be honest I only really focussed on the last paragraph which said, *"It is normal to worry when you are urgently referred to see a specialist by your GP, nurse, or dentist. However, more than nine out of every ten people referred this way will not be diagnosed with cancer"*. So there was nothing to be concerned about was there? I even put the appointment back a week to fit in a holiday we had booked.

I went to my appointment at the head and neck clinic of the hospital on my own, thinking it was just a routine check-up. A camera was sent up my nose to examine the back of my throat and it was while I was blowing my nose and wiping the watery eyes caused by this, I asked the consultant what he thought. His reply did not really sink in at first: he said a biopsy was needed to confirm, but if I allowed him an educated guess, he thought I had a cancerous tumour. If I allowed him a further educated guess, it was eminently treatable. I had to then go immediately for a pre-assessment and fill in a consent form for the biopsy that was to be done within forty-eight hours. I remember walking around Leeds city centre in a daze not knowing what to think, but it was slowly and belatedly dawning on me that I was in trouble.

I went home and waited for my wife to return from work to give her the news, not an easy conversation as I really did not know what to think myself. We talked it through and decided to keep it to ourselves until we knew for certain, taking hope from the consultant's last comment of a successful treatment being the most likely outcome.

The biopsy confirmed I had a squamous cell carcinoma affecting the base of my tongue, tonsils and neck that was caused by the HPV virus, the one children are now being vaccinated against. Probably because of my lack of action earlier, the tumour was too big to remove surgically, so a treatment of two doses of chemotherapy and seven weeks of radiotherapy were prescribed.

It was all a whirlwind of appointments from then on: a mask made for radiotherapy treatment, CT scans, dentist checks, even speech therapy boot-camp sessions all within two or three weeks. My GP said the treatment would be gruelling. He was not wrong and I got to understand the true meaning of the word.

It was a long seven weeks and in the last few weeks I was finding it increasingly difficult to eat and drink, but I got through to the last treatment session at the end of November and rang the celebratory bell, glad it was all over. Unfortunately, radiotherapy has a cumulative effect and within a few days of finishing treatment I was admitted to hospital severely dehydrated and three stone lighter! A feeding tube was inserted that I had for four weeks until it was removed on the 30th of December. What an unexpected year 2017 turned out to be!

Happily, three months later I got the all clear from the consultant so with the support of my wife, family, friends and people at work I had beaten it! The only lasting side effects were a little scarring to my neck from the radiotherapy and reduced saliva production, making eating dry foods difficult without sipping lots of water—try eating three cream crackers one after another without drinking anything to understand what I mean).

I felt fit and well and, at the insistence of my family, it was decided I should try and give something back for all the support and excellent service I had received from the NHS. So on behalf of the Leeds Cares charity, we did a fundraising walk in September 2019 doing the Yorkshire Three Peaks Challenge and between us raised over £6,000. It was two proud days, first to successfully do the walk with all my family and friends around me and then to present the cheque at Bexley Wing, St James's hospital.

Raising the money also gave me closure on my cancer journey. I had kept a positive attitude throughout and never lost hope. I was in very capable hands and was lucky to have the support from everyone I knew. So that was it, done and dusted.

Soon after this, news started to be heard of a strange virus emanating from China, and we all know what happened then!

It was early in 2021 during lockdown that I started feeling strange pains in my left leg and over the weeks found it uncomfortable to stand and walk for long periods. I saw my doctor who suspected sciatica and referred me for physiotherapy. I was given an exercise regime which did not seem to help. I paid for chiropractor sessions that included acupuncture and massages but it just got worse.

I was eventually sent for an MRI scan on my back one Sunday. I was totally convinced it was just a disc in my vertebrae that was pressing on my sciatic nerve, the classic cause of sciatica, so again was not really too concerned. However, I immediately knew I was in trouble when the technician who was operating the MRI machine stopped me as I was leaving. They asked if I had ever experienced my foot dropping at all or any numbness in my back passage and that if I did, I was immediately to go to A&E. Very alarming as nothing was normally said after the scans I had in the past.

The phone call I got at work the following day from my GP was devastating. *"I am sorry, Mister Hollingworth, but we think it is a cancerous tumour in your spine."* Covid was still around and telephone appointments were the norm, but this is not the way you want to have this sort of news delivered.

Another biopsy followed to confirm that the cancer I'd had before had returned, but this time it had spread to other parts of my body—pelvis and ribs—and worse still, it could not be cured and that any treatment would be palliative only. I am told it is unusual for this type of cancer to return and that I have been unlucky. The comment at the time was that they don't know what the future holds for me!

This was tough to process and a lot of dark thoughts followed in the fog of uncertainty, and at times I felt little hope. I also had an initial mis-diagnosis of myeloma which did not help. The excellent oncologist I had in 2017 had left, and it would be fair to say his replacement did not have the same empathy or communication skills. On the positive side, I had five sessions of radiotherapy to my spine and very soon after, the debilitating sciatica was gone!

I was also supposed to start chemotherapy treatment in January 2022 but follow up CT scans showed that the other tumours were very small and had not changed much, so this was deferred until the benefits of the treatment outweighed the chemotherapy side effects.

I am pleased to say I now have a new oncologist who I am very happy with. My last scan has shown further small lesions in my lungs and liver so at the time of writing, my treatment has commenced and I am now halfway through six cycles of chemotherapy over an eighteen-week period. Already I have had some positive news, in that my blood tests have shown some indication that the treatment appears to be working.

Other than the sciatica I suffered with last year, my cancer has been completely asymptomatic with no pain or illness thankfully. I now have a very positive oncologist who has explained this is just one of many treatments in her armoury and that, although the cancer has been spreading, the tumours are very small and have been caught early, so I am hopeful that my cancer can be managed for many years to come. I feel so lucky to have such a supportive family, friends and workplace, not something everyone is blessed with I know.

I will always be optimistic, for me and for the sake of my wife and two sons, remaining ever hopeful. The opposite of hopefulness to me would be despair, and that cannot, and will not, enter into my thoughts.

Ian Hollingworth

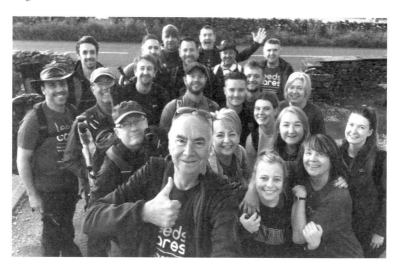

Big Boys Don't Cry

I HAVE BEEN CHARGED AT BY ALL BLACKS AND FIJIAN JUGGERNAUTS and come round to the aroma of smelling salts, with a different profile on a few occasions. My speed and guile helped me to dodge many a broken bone but this was a tackle I couldn't swerve.

No rub down, no clunks from a chiropractor or deep tissue massage would help with this one. This was a deeper heat. Sport, and a successful sales career, had taken me all over the world but 2014 had other plans.

My younger brother Stuart (or *"Tut Stu"* as he was nicknamed by the yachting community in the Antibes, due to his Yorkshire accent and habit of saying *"I'm going t'shop or t'pub"*) had more stamps on his passport than James Bond.

As a deck hand on executive yachts, he'd crewed several round-the-world tours in spite of getting seasick. Stus' offices included Antibes, the Caribbean and Sri Lanka. He had seen places many only dream of, living a life some considered a myth.

Stu had a very private side to him which only close family and friends experienced. He was half-health food, half-hedonism, working hard all day to party all night. Whilst others burnt the candle at both ends, he sometimes would take a flamethrower to his—he was never going to be a slow-burner.

Stu was on the other side of the world in Thailand, complaining of back aches and pain in his legs. After a few months of typical male stubbornness and losing his balance for the second time in a month, he was eventually persuaded to see a doctor at a private clinic. The hospital initially diagnosed him with DVT (deep vein thrombosis) and Warfarin was prescribed. Unfortunately, they gave him too much, which resulted in Stu experiencing internal bleeding. This meant they did more tests and took more pictures and scans. They didn't like the look of the results on camera so Stuart was advised to seek further help immediately at another hospital.

A few days later my middle brother, David, who lived in Eastleigh, received a phone call from his girlfriend in Thailand—she was acting as an interpreter for Stuart at the hospital – saying Stuart had had his spleen and thirty percent of his stomach removed.

He called me immediately to relay this information. I remember I put my pint of beer on the table in the pub where I was watching the World Cup group game of Italy v Costa Rica, who were in England's group—funny how you remember these minute details—and told him I would make plans to leave on the earliest flight. I would bring mum with me; I knew she would want to be there, and I knew Stuart would have wanted her there as well. You never realise how much you need your mum until you're ill on the other side of the planet; he needed mum—urgently.

I told her we were going out to see him to lift his spirits, because he was poorly, and to check everything was okay. I booked business class, to make it look more of a treat, as I genuinely thought we would only be there a week at the most and mum had never 'turned left' on a long-haul flight before.

At this point we were all clinging onto the hope that whatever he had was treatable or curable. Stu was young and extremely fit; surely if we got him the right help, he would beat whatever it was that was wrong with him?

We were due to leave York by train the next day to catch a flight to Bangkok from Heathrow. An hour before we met up at the station, David called me again to update me on Stuart's condition. He told me that the results from the scans had showed Stuart had pancreatic cancer, that it had spread, and his condition was terminal. We both agreed I wouldn't tell mum until we reached the hospital in Pattaya the following day.

For eighteen hours, I had to lie—well, not tell the truth to a woman I adored. I had to protect the woman who had always protected us.

It seemed like a lifetime. There was nowhere to hide from the expert interrogator sitting opposite me; she could read me like a book, but I couldn't, and wouldn't, tell her the truth. She had said *"goodbye"* to too many people who had made her happy in recent times: her mother, who was the centre of our family, the matriarch we looked up to, every Saturday smothered in grandchildren. Her second husband Albert, who we all loved dearly and years earlier her nephew, Phillip, who only reached his late twenties.

We reached a suburb of Pattaya and entered the local district hospital. It wasn't the most clinical hospital in the world—Stuart hadn't renewed his health insurance but never told us—and never have I missed the NHS more. This was only a few rungs above spit-and-sawdust, with families sleeping in hallways, very basic conditions and very noisy, but, despite this, the nurses were amazing.

I was about to tell mum the real truth about his diagnosis of stage four pancreatic cancer just before we were due to see him in the ward. We were walking down the corridor to the ward and I stopped her, sat her on a bench and started to tell her. And that is when she said she knew.

Mums know. They just do. It's their job to protect you at whatever age. No matter how big and ugly, you're still their little boy. She understood.

Seeing Stuart and knowing the dire situation he was in, our hope had transferred from saving him, to getting him home to be with his family and friends. Stuart had spent the first twenty-five years of his life in York and we all wanted him home.

We hoped that there was time to do this.

They day after we landed, the surgeon confirmed to us, face-to-face, that Stuart had been diagnosed with stage four pancreatic cancer and there was no chance of long-term survival. It's a weird thing, but I really hoped, and prayed, it would make him pass away quickly. This is the dark side of hope and I've carried the guilt of this thought for eight years. I didn't want my brother to suffer and for his death to be drawn out.

I stayed for a week, as it was agreed my role was to work on a plan to fly my brother back home, no matter what. This needed a lot of research as well as financial management back home in York.

My mother stayed for over four weeks and made the best of a terrible situation. She astonished us in how she handled and managed everything and, with the help and support of my middle brother David and his girlfriend who had also flown out a few days after me, they tried to comfort and nurse Stuart as he gradually deteriorated and grew weaker.

Everyone thinks I'm a big strong man but at every stage I've been surrounded by even stronger women, an array of mothers and aunties plus a wife who exceed their constituent parts.

We had to get Stuart home. It wasn't going to be easy—the cost was astronomical!—but money soon lost all value. The exchange rate and figures on a statement became meaningless as his need grew greater. Nothing else mattered.

Stu could only leave once the consultant at the hospital had assessed him and given the okay that he was 'fit to fly'. They gave him the green light and with all logistics organised, we got him back to England. The ambulance was waiting on the runway and with oxygen masks in place—next stop York district hospital. Home James, and don't spare the horses. The clock was ticking.

Once Stuart was back in York, I walked into his room and was physically shocked to see how far he had deteriorated since I last saw him. He was losing his voice, and he was so weak, but he still smiled and gave us a thumbs up. This was just a few weeks since I'd seen him in Thailand.

My overriding hope at that point for him, was that he would slip away soon.

I never shared this hope with anyone until I was asked to share my story for this book and I have carried the guilt of my feelings ever since.

The registrar explained that the medical team had already started running tests on Stu's condition and he would update us once the results were available. Just over an hour later we were shown to a private room where mum and I were told by the senior consultant, *"Your son is seriously ill and won't last the night."*

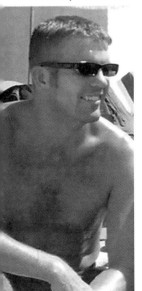

We were so thankful for their honesty. There were no breakdowns, no floods of tears. Mum said I had to get our dad here quickly, and also mum's army of sisters. Most them worked or had worked in the NHS or in care services and were a fantastic support over the next few hours.

Mum and dad hadn't really spoken more than a few words for years due to dad's attitude even though he, by his own admission, had not been the ideal husband in the later years of their marriage. Mum had remarried and had been very happy.

When dad arrived he was brilliant with mum; all his previous bitterness had left him and genuine love and warmth was evident to everyone in the room, reminding me of a Christmas football match in a First World War no-man's land.

He held mum's hand and simply said, *"Thank you for looking after my son. You've done a fantastic job."*

At 6.35pm, just six hours after arriving back in York, our homing pigeon left us for good. Did he wait for us all to be there? Why did

Stu Mercer

87

it take something so horrific to get dad talking with sincerity and respect to mum again? Was it his gift to all of us?

Once Stuart had left us, it was an immense relief to me that he didn't suffer and was at peace, and I had got what I had guiltily hoped for.

At the funeral, dad—now in a wheelchair—got to his feet and patted the coffin. The room fell silent. In the days, weeks and months that followed my mum and dad continued to speak to each other on a regular basis with my mum helping my auntie Helen, alongside my other aunts, to care for dad until he too passed away, the following January, just six months after Stu. My brother Dave and I believe that Stu's passing away broke his heart and that was the real beginning of his decline in health.

Stuart died with just a large sports kit bag to show for four decades on the planet. He made it and blew it! Lassies loved him. They described him as *a bloke to go shopping with, who would give you his last penny.* He saw more of the world than most do in a lifetime. He crammed eighty-six years into forty-six. He lived fast—perhaps too fast. He lived the highest of the high lives, always washed down with a glass of champagne. He had a shy and vulnerable side to him, but most only saw his more rock 'n' roll exterior.

Could I have done more to help him?

Do I feel guilty for wanting him to die?

I've got to stop this.

I have a photo of his enormous scar from surgery—it seems odd to everyone else, but it was part of him.

I have identical photos of Stuart and dad at the races—happy together and full of life—in both my lounge and my office. I don't know anyone else with the same photo in two rooms of their house, but it helps me. I see them as I always want to see them—like I said, happy together and full of life.

Dave is still the middle one; nothing changed there and we're closer than ever before because of this tragic event.

But so much has changed since then...

Material things mean little today; they don't make me happy.

I used to value money; now I value time and people.

Julie, my wife, is invaluable, somehow always knowing when to help and when to leave me alone, to just get on with it.

I hope I am still good company, and I still meet the boys for a pint to watch the footy or rugby. I still love a good party and I still love life.

A dear friend has instilled into me the motto *"Life is too short"* and this has become my mantra, and it gives me hope.

Apparently big boys don't cry.

Well, I cry every day. I've never told anyone this before.

I don't think I'm alone.

It helps.

Andy Mercer *(Credit Ian Donaghy)*

Finding Hope in the Darkness

FOR AS LONG AS I CAN REMEMBER I have had a bump on the lower part of my neck. However, one evening my wife, Fay, looked at me curiously and said, *"What's that—it looks a bit odd?"* I assured her it had been there since… forever, but as a precaution I visited the doctor at my office. Following a short examination, the doctor confidently stated it was a harmless fatty lump and advised that it would be a simple cosmetic procedure to have it removed. Job done, or maybe not!

Given the apparent lack of urgency, I made an appointment with my local GP to discuss the removal. In the interim, I noticed a smaller lump at the top of my neck. I passed the GP a letter from the doctor who had assured me it should be a simple cosmetic procedure. The GP did not share this view and proceeded to make a follow up referral with the Ear, Nose and Throat (ENT) Team, ending my appointment with the phrase, *"I'll ask them to rush it"*.

When I met the ENT consultant at Kirkcaldy Victoria Hospital, I again enthusiastically explained the original view of a cosmetic procedure and brandished my letter like a shield. The consultant moved quickly to discount the original diagnosis, used uncomfortable scopes to examine my throat, and fired requests at colleagues about the need for urgent follow up appointments. It was then he uttered the phrase *"potentially cancerous"*. I vividly remember feeling a horrible sinking sensation as the world start to spin away from me and I no longer felt in control. When I got home, I was shaken and explained to Fay what had happened. Over the next few weeks, I tried to keep calm as nothing had yet been confirmed. Relatives with previous medical experience played things down and said it was standard for doctors to caution that lumps could be cancerous.

The next step was a neck biopsy at Dunfermline's Queen Margaret Hospital. It felt like the man who completed the procedure used a spade as it really hurt. Strangely, he had been directed only to biopsy the smaller lump at the top of my neck. When I asked about the original larger bump, he dismissed it is a simple cyst and continued his digging.

It took a couple of weeks for the results. At that point I learned a big lesson; waiting is one of the worst parts. Unfortunately, the results proved inconclusive; there were signs of potential anomalies, but the analysis team were *"not sure"*. I was declared a medical mystery. In the world of ENT, cancer always travels downwards whereas my lumps had moved up from the base of my neck. The consultant appeared optimistic it could be something simple, but in the interim referred me to Edinburgh Cancer Care Centre.

The first time I entered the centre was very intimidating. On arrival you are issued with a repeat appointment card. I had it in my head this was a one-off, I'm not sick, I didn't belong in here—it was all a big misunderstanding! When my name was called, I took a deep breath before being taken to meet the consultation team. My results had been reviewed but they weren't sure. More tests! A second biopsy this time at Lauriston Place in Edinburgh. We left with polite thanks, my appointment card marked, and the sinking feeling.

The doctor who completed the second biopsy was genuinely kind and supportive. After my initial experience I was nervous, and he was shocked the first biopsy had completed without anaesthetic. He was very experienced and when I asked for his view he nodded slowly and said there was a very high probability it was cancer (cautioning the result were subject to lab analysis). He recognised this was a difficult message and urged I should take time to contemplate the news. I headed to the canteen and felt that sinking feeling again. I tried to *"keep calm and carry on"* and worked from home in the afternoon. I remember being on the phone when my biopsy wound reopened with blood pouring onto my work pad. Stupid.

Again, more waiting as the results were processed then another trip to Edinburgh Cancer Care Centre. This time there was no doubt it was cancer: metastatic melanoma. This was why it had travelled up rather than down. It's highly aggressive and would kill me if left untreated. This was one of my lowest points. That evening we shared the news with the children (ages six and eight) dad was ill with a condition called cancer. They were curious and asked great questions, *"Will you die, Daddy?"*, *"Can we still hug you?"* Many tears and hugs.

Despite a questionable emotional state, I again tried the *"keep calm and carry on"* approach and headed to work the next day and again it didn't work out well. I ended up breaking down in a station toilet being comforted by a friend and colleague. With the benefit of hindsight, I was in denial and trying to protect myself by clinging to a rock of normality.

The consultants were unsure where the cancer had originated and how far it had spread. Despite being melanoma there were never any visible signs on the skin with things triggering internally. More tests, more waiting. CT scans, PET scans, dermatology examinations. Having been diagnosed and seeing the condition of others at the Edinburgh centre I fought with difficult thoughts, and I wondered how deep this pit would go.

Through my journey I found hope an easy thing to lose and a hard thing to recover. Moving through the diagnosis stage was particularly tough, the 'clinical' direct nature of the medical teams was understandable but brutal. Each new appointment seemed to bring more bad news, quickly eroding the hope I had held onto. A huge cliché, but through the most difficult of times it was thoughts of my children which provided the hope and determination to fight and keep pushing forwards.

Back to Edinburgh for the results. The scans and investigations confirmed the tumours were in my neck, however, did not appear to have spread further with the lymph nodes having done their job—a glimmer of optimism, but time was critical.

My treatment plan was to be split into two stages: a full neck dissection followed by radiotherapy (chemo has no impact on melanoma). The consultant was very clear the treatment would be testing; however the talk of treatment was a small, but real, source of hope and from that point forward it was important I trusted in the process.

After what felt like month—but in reality, was a couple of weeks—a date for the operation was confirmed and shortly afterward the day arrived. We drove to the hospital early and walked up to the ENT ward. Having had very little experience of hospital wards it was a daunting experience. Throat cancers typically affect older men as a result the ward was full of older gentlemen with massive trauma to their throats. Time to be brave.

The surgery was complex and lasted seven hours. I was in hospital for five days and the immediate recovery period was hard. I had three drainage tubes and a large stapled wound, running from ear to chest. The simplest tasks—taking a shower, going to the toilet—were tricky, but one by one the drains were removed and to great relief I got home, and my wounds began to heal. The world normalised for a month or so and then I returned to Edinburgh to discuss the next phase of the treatment plan.

Although I had heard of radiotherapy, I knew little about how it worked and the effects. My oncologist began with an overview of radiotherapy and even managed to throw in a bit of radiotherapy humour (jokes about not becoming the Incredible Hulk). Given the aggressive nature of the condition a six-week daily schedule of treatment was prescribed. The oncologist stepped us through the plan, highlighting the significant and painful side effects. I was put on a high fat diet and instructed to consume as many calories as possible because the burning effect of the radiotherapy would make it difficult to eat and could result in significant weight loss. Not all bad I guess, but cakes didn't taste as good when being eaten for medicinal purposes.

In readiness for the radiotherapy, I was fitted with a plastic mask. The mask, which was very, very uncomfortable, was needed to immobilise me ensuring the radiation was targeted with pinpoint accuracy. Additionally I had four teeth extracted for good measure to minimise the requirement for future dental work.

And so, day one of the radiotherapy arrived. The senior nurse gave me a formal welcome and introduced me to her team. She recapped the horrible side effects then armed me with a huge tub of sterile smelling moisturising emollient cream and advised me to gargle with baking powder to try and relieve the pain. And so that was me set, every day for six weeks. Because it spanned Christmas and New Year I was hit twice a day on a couple of occasions. The first couple of weeks were okay but moving into week three the treatment began to kick. It was a very gruelling period. Thankfully I managed to keep eating although my diet was very limited. Head down, session by session, week by week the treatment was ticked off and in the second week of January my treatment plan was completed. Toward the end of January, I met with the consultants at the Edinburgh Cancer Care Centre and dared ask the question what next? "That's it," was the reply and I was returned to care at my local hospital.

Since then there have been scares and setbacks, but I am on the journey of recovery living my life in ever longer time horizons rather than being unable to see past the next appointment. Other than my family and the medical services to both of whom I owe my life, the strongest support has come from Maggies. The team at Kirkcaldy helped me properly reflect and process what had happened. Despite being scared, the team have helped me to find renewed hope and move forward toward a new normal where life's priorities have been redrawn, although I am now a hypochondriac!

Graeme Macgregor

Receiving a Terminal Bowel Cancer Diagnosis Saved My Life

IN **MARCH 2016 I REINSTATED MY DATING PROFILE ON TINDER** after helping a work colleague get to the point where guys actually wanted to have a discussion with her, rather than something casual. It had been three years since I'd been emotionally battered by a tricky divorce, when I fought for sanity and the right to be treated with respect and compassion from those who had been used to me being a 'people pleaser'.

I met Russ as soon as I uploaded my profile and he, too, wanted to have a two-way chat. Radical! We met, hit it off and spent the next six months dating—without children hanging around our ankles wanting our attention. In November 2016 we decided to rent a house together. Quick? Yes! I can still hear my mum's concerned words, *"He seems great, but do you think it would be better to get to know each other more?"* But it felt right. I rented out my house so that I had something to fall back on if we didn't work out.

That Christmas was the first time I felt like myself for a long time. I often looked around at the new people and stepchildren in my life, wondering how life could get better? I felt that after a mentally and physically testing time everything had eventually come to a place of harmony. We were a good team. A good parenting team. A good couple. We were happy to have found each other. We became 'The Secret Seven'—a blended family.

I had been working part-time for an events company. My boss was demanding, shouty and pushy. I felt torn between telling him to get lost, and feeling appreciative to have a job that fitted around my two young children. I began dreading going into the office. One morning I remember developing a rash on my chest. I put it down to a virus. I made frequent trips to the toilet to cry because I didn't have the skills and confidence to stand up to my boss. I lost my voice. Over a period of around six–nine months, I ignored the blood I was passing in my stools. It was just haemorrhoids, a payback from spending three days in labour and then having two emergency c-sections, surely?

I was fit, healthy, went to the gym, loved broccoli, chickpeas, fresh food, and drank lots of water. Tick, tick, tick. Nothing could be wrong with me.

However, between Christmas and New Year, Russ and I went away. I remember looking down into the toilet and seeing the bright red blood. No pain, no straining, just blood and a lot of it. It scared me. I couldn't ignore it any more.

I booked an appointment with my GP, went along and talked about my moods. I chickened out. I booked another appointment and cancelled it because the bleeding was inconsistent. There were days when everything was normal. At last I plucked up the courage to have the conversation. I mentioned that my mum has ulcerative colitis and it was this that triggered him to invite me to have a colonoscopy. Not really the kind of invite you ever want to receive, but it turned into a life-destroying/saving moment.

Two weeks later, being supported by my best buddy, I endured drinking the liquid they give you to clear your system. No amount of orange squash changes the taste to something that's pleasant, but it's essential. For the sake of a moment of time that's uncomfortable, you really have to dig deep and go with the flow (literally).

Lying down, looking at the screen, and seeing my insides was fascinating, albeit a little like something out of a sci-fi movie. After a lot of wiggling around, the tone and whole atmosphere dropped. I remember the guy who was performing the colonoscopy saying, *"Oh, can you see this?"* He was prodding something that didn't look very happy. It was red and bulgy. He asked if he could tattoo my insides. Result—my first tattoo, ever.

We sat with him afterwards and he explained that this angry lump needed investigation. I went numb, sitting there stoically thinking that I should've gone earlier to see my GP. I beat myself up for being a plonker for not acting on what my body was screaming and trying to tell me.

Fast-forward a couple of weeks after a multitude of CT scans and MRIs and wondering what the heck was going on. This wasn't right, I looked after myself. My time for being ill wasn't now. Bowel cancer is for older people who love sausage rolls, beer and smoking. Not me—the person who can hold a headstand for minutes on end, a trained yoga teacher who is calm and contained.

We were invited to receive the results of all the scans and the biopsy with the consultant. My mum joined me and Russ. The cancer nurse opened the room and locked the door after her. That's never a good sign, is it?

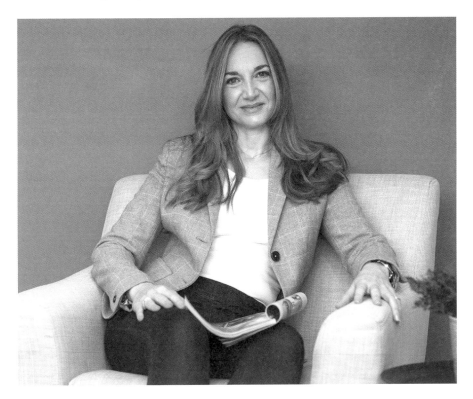

The consultant, the person who had performed my colonoscopy, gave us the news. The cancer had spread to my liver and lungs. There was nothing they could do apart from offer me palliative care. We cried in the room next door to the consultant. We went back to my friend's house and drank a lot of bubbles, pinching ourselves to wake up from the nightmare that was real.

We told the kids. They were aged six to thirteen years at the time. I didn't want them not knowing. We told them in the most appropriate way we could. I can't remember the words. I cried buckets. We considered second opinions and clinics in Europe, claiming miraculous recovery. I talked to Macmillan and made the most of their services and specialist nurses.

All of my friends and family visited often. I received more cards than the shelves at Clintons.

For two weeks I planned my funeral, spent time with people, blamed myself for eating bacon rolls, cursed myself for not being strong enough through a tricky divorce.

People talk about the injustice and unfairness of cancer and I never knew what they meant until then. I am the one who loves Mediterranean food, avoids junk, avoids boozing, etc. *"Why is this happening to me?"* became my inner dialogue.

After this very human period of blame, I decided to work out what I could do to help myself. My inner dialogue and belief became *"I'm going to live!"* This was the first glimmer of hope.

I'd been through such a testing time for two years during my divorce that I decided that this was not my time to depart this earth. I had so much to live for. My family, my new relationship, real happiness and love. I wasn't ready to let it go.

I researched additional ways I could help myself. I didn't believe it when my consultant said, *"Eat what you like"*. Surely food is medicine, right? In my mind, I told myself that I'd created it, and therefore I can uncreate it. That's quite strong isn't it? By the way, I no longer tell myself that I created it because that wouldn't be helpful.

I didn't want to fight cancer, to beat it. I wanted to work with my body and mind. Why would I want to be at war with my whole self? It didn't make sense. I told myself that my cells were 'confused' and they needed time to work out a different way to get better.

Then, everything changed. A couple of weeks after, the original terminal diagnosis changed, allowing me to have surgery and chemo. Everyone was up in arms. *"How could they get it sooooo wrong?"*

When the scans had been re-examined and shared with multiple professionals, it transpired that although I did have lung nodules they were too small to categorise. I did have activity in my liver but it was blood vessels not the cancer spreading. All of this positive news enabled me to be offered the opportunity to have an operation to remove the tumour. Funnily enough, I had enjoyed previous stays in hospital when I was young. The insertion of a grommet for the fixing of a hearing issue when I was young. The insertion of a metal plate in my arm when I fell from the climbing apparatus in PE, a tonsillectomy in my twenties, two emergency c-sections with my children, so the thought of being on the operating table was liberating, rather than fear-inducing.

I accepted that things were going in a different direction. This was my chance. I had to sit up, take notice and change how I was living. Hope grew and built up from the inside out.

I dismissed the emails from people wanting to sell me magic juice diets and retreats. I tweaked my diet, visited a reputable homoeopath, had regular reflexology and focused on nourishing my whole system.

I took six weeks off after surgery. The resection went brilliantly. I was fortunate not to have a stoma. Recovery was good. I went back to work. Results from the lymph nodes put another spanner in my plans. They showed I was at stage three. I had no idea what this meant, but I remember receiving the call stating that I would be offered chemo.

My hair! I've had long hair forever! It's a huge part of me. No no no.

After accepting this next step and receiving everyone else's opinions, I decided to go for it. I had to be flexible and dig deep with my sense of hope. I had to give myself the best chance of survival.

After six months I received the 'all-clear'. And that's when I fell apart. Doesn't sound right, does it? But the therapist told me that this is when she sees the majority of her clients—when they realise their life is limited.

One of the problems when you get the 'all-clear' from cancer is that everyone expects you to be jumping for joy and 'back to normal'. You don't. It takes time to unravel everything. It's messy. It's pushing people away when you need them the most. It's not telling people how you feel because you just can't pick the words. It's the memory of receiving the call to tell you that you're at stage 3, when you have no idea what that means but you can tell from the tone of voice that your days are numbered. It's the physical exhaustion allowing your body to recover from surgery and chemo. It's the remembering of how painful chemo really is.

It feels like everything doesn't really matter anymore.

It feels like everything matters.

It's like being ultra-sensitive and fearless all in one.

It's a mindf@ck.

Yes, I still have moments when I don't cope well. Yes, I'm not a robot. No, I'm not brave. No, I don't have all the answers. Yes, talking is imperative. It's a non-negotiable.

After end-of-life counselling I managed to pick myself back up again. I worked out what I should be focusing on. For me, it was the ability to use my voice. To ask for what I needed. To achieve meaningful work. To be a parent whom the kids could always talk to. To put my self-care first. I found out who I was and everyday I'm enjoying exploring my capabilities.

I guess I fired up that 'rebellious hope'!

I love firing up other people's rebellious hope, especially those who are going through life-changing diagnosis.

Cancer saved my life. I'm grateful for the chance to look death in the eye and say *"No, not yet"*.

Tasha Thor-Straten

Not Just Skin Cancer

AS A FAMILY, WE ONLY WENT ON HOLIDAY FOR TWO WEEKS EVERY YEAR and never abroad. In the Seventies, the only 'sunscreen' available was tanning oil—used to enhance a tan! I should also mention that I did use a sun bed three times but only for a very short period—fifteen minutes—per session. As I grew older, I didn't consider myself at particularly high risk of skin cancer due to so little exposure to the sun and only in the UK. How wrong I was!

I've had a large area of flat, pigmented skin at the back of my lower left leg (the size of a ginger nut biscuit) since I was around ten years old. Over the years, when more became known about the dangers of the sun, I had this pigmented area checked occasionally and there was never any problem. I also used a high factor sunscreen as they were becoming more readily available. My GP had checked the pigmented area early in 2016 and whilst he wasn't concerned, he did tell me to continue to come and have it checked more regularly. It is now known that melanoma can take many years to surface. Life was busy and unfortunately I didn't go to see him until April 2017 to check on a small rough patch that had developed with the pigmented area—that was probably my biggest mistake.

I was referred to the dermatology unit at my local hospital and I had a biopsy which confirmed malignant melanoma—a huge shock. An operation followed. This procedure needed a large skin graft and this was followed by a second operation as it was decided not enough healthy skin had been taken from around the melanoma site. The skin graft took many months to completely heal, and I have been left with a large hole at the back of my leg and lymphedema.

Three monthly scans and skin checks followed, and all was well until early 2020, just as the Covid-19 pandemic struck. I developed a lump on the shin of my left leg. It was hot and painful and on a visit to the GP, where I was seen by a paramedic (the GP surgery was short staffed), I was treated for cellulitis and given antibiotics and cream. Fortunately, I also had an appointment for a skin check a few days later. The CNS (Clinical Nurse Specialist) wasn't happy with the lump and immediately referred me back to hospital to be seen by the oncology team. Once again, my life was turned upside down as I was told this was a return of the melanoma and there were also smaller lumps around my ankle. I believe this is referred to as 'In Transit Melanoma'. Being situated on my shin, the lump was considered too difficult to remove surgically as it would require another extensive skin graft, but the oncology team knew of a trial being performed at the Royal Marsden cancer hospital in London. I agreed to take this option and was accepted. This gave me hope as the procedure is designed to kill off cancer in limbs and I was fortunate at that time to not have any further spread within my body.

The trial (called the Titan Trial) involved injecting the main lump (tumour) in my leg with a drug called T-Vec. T-Vec teaches your immune system to destroy cancer cells but usually only acts on 'local' areas and not throughout your body. I was injected with this drug on two occasions, three weeks apart at the Royal Marsden. All cancer drugs can cause side effects. I certainly had some following the T-Vec injections, but they were manageable. I then had a major operation called an Isolated Limb Perfusion. This was a six–seven hour procedure where the circulation in the affected leg was cut off and my leg flushed with an extremely high dose of chemicals to kill off the tumour. I was also given a third T-Vec injection. I had all the lymph nodes in my groin removed which caused further leg swelling. After a six day stay in hospital I returned home to recover completely. It took some time and I had to regain the ability to walk properly, slowly over a few weeks. Eventually though, I was okay and able to carry on with life, although not able to walk as far as I once could. I also found (and still do) kneeling and getting up off the floor difficult.

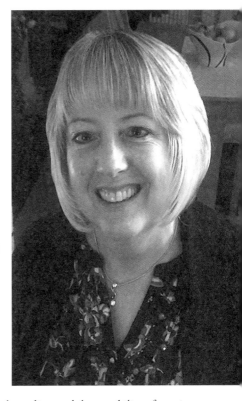

Then followed a year of scans and follow up appointments at the Royal Marsden, where I was eventually advised that the tumours in my leg had all but disappeared and the large one was not detectable on scans. The trial procedure had worked for me. I was elated. My consultant said I'd had an amazing response and that he would like to keep following me up. He also said he wouldn't discharge me from the hospital as a patient as I could ask to be referred back to them in the future—something I later needed to take advantage of, although I didn't know it at the time!

I had my final scans in July 2021 at Royal Marsden and thought all would be well. How wrong I was! I received a phone call to say that an abnormality had showed up near my duodenum that needed investigating. Royal Marsden wanted to carry out the required biopsies and this was done in early September. Unfortunately, it was a melanoma tumour. I was now classed as stage four as the cancer had moved to an organ. The consultant discussed the possibility of a major operation to remove my duodenum and part of my pancreas, called a 'Whipple operation'. This procedure is generally only carried out in a few major cancer centres and is not offered as the first course of action for melanoma tumours.

I was instead offered immunotherapy. This is where you are given infusions of powerful drugs to 'teach' your immune system to destroy cancer cells – it is a little more complex than that and the science is amazing. I opted for this, and it was agreed that I could have the infusions at my local hospital. After a consultation with a medical oncologist, treatment started at the beginning of November 2021. I was given the combination known as Ipi/Nivo, which had been hailed as a 'miracle' drug, so I was very hopeful that this would work for me.

All seemed to go well with fatigue and an itchy rash being the only side effects—I had been given a booklet which listed all the possible side effects, some very severe, but I hoped I wouldn't experience them. Unfortunately, after two cycles of the drugs I developed severe colitis, a common side effect of immunotherapy, and I had to be treated with steroids. Initially, the steroids didn't help so I was hospitalised twice, at two different hospitals.

Immunotherapy can work very well but it doesn't work for everyone and can cause severe side effects. My treatment was halted because of my adverse reaction to the drugs, which included my liver being affected, but I thought that once all this had been resolved, treatment would be re-started using another drug with less toxicity.

How wrong I was, again!

Following my discharge from my local hospital, I continued to take the medication I had been prescribed. My colitis cleared up quickly and my liver started to return to normal. I was originally told that the tumour had started to shrink a little. By the end of March 2022, I knew I needed help in managing the stomach pains so I was advised to go to a different hospital where I was given ibuprofen—what a relief, the pain disappeared. I also had scans to check my abdomen for blockage or any other abnormalities.

I then received a request to go over to my local hospital at the end of that week to discuss my recent scan. I wasn't asked to bring anyone with me so I went alone as I would normally have done. I was called into a consulting room and told that my tumour had increased in size and was now in the head of my pancreas. I asked what would happen next.

Little did I know that the bottom was about to drop out of my world again! I was told that the immunotherapy hadn't worked and there was no other treatment they could offer. I felt that hope had been taken from me, and I was all alone.

My husband was called to come to the hospital to be told this news. Following the expected 'meltdown' I had, I remembered my Royal Marsden consultant's words and asked for a referral back to them. I know they can offer treatments that many other hospitals don't have access to—including the 'Whipple' procedure.

The referral was made a few days after the consultation, and I was also advised that a referral had been made to another hospital near-by, which has a more specialist cancer centre and can often treat complex cases. I don't know why this option wasn't discussed with me during my consultation—it might have given me a little hope, which is extremely important when you are battling any sort of cancer.

The Royal Marsden decided that they didn't recommend the 'Whipple' procedure due to one of my veins being 'draped' over the tumour. Also, although they had a Phase 1 trial, I wasn't eligible to take part because of the adverse effects I had recently experienced. I was extremely disappointed—I really thought the experts there might have been able to help me, and hope again disappeared.

I then decided to carry out my own research into treatments and trials being carried out all over the country. I joined the Facebook group 'Melanomamates' and used the Melanoma UK and Melanoma Focus websites. The information and experiences of others in similar situations to me, gave me the hope and confidence to ask questions and challenge the doctors.

With the help of Gill Nuttall, CEO of Melanoma UK, I was able to have an informed discussion with my oncologist to put forward various options which we explored, and he agreed there were options to investigate and I had not reached the end of the road.

Being prepared for this meeting was vital to my hope index.

I have now started a new round of immunotherapy treatment, and I have hope that this treatment will help me, and I also hope and believe that there are other treatments becoming available that will prove successful and with more manageable side effects... and that I will be able to benefit from them.

On my cancer journey I have experienced different levels of care and advice, and I would advise anyone in a similar situation to make sure that if a hospital, or your local health authority, can't help anymore that you are advised you can make their own enquiries on trials and other treatments, and seek another opinion.

I sincerely hope that you are given options, and I hope you don't leave hearing they have nothing left to offer you.

Dianne Butler

Cancer can be a Drama

WHEN I GOT CANCER EIGHTEEN YEARS AGO AT THE AGE OF THIRTY-NINE, there wasn't a lot of information available to me and my family on what was to come and how to deal with it. I considered myself to be quite fit, as I was playing football twice a week as well as kicking the ball around regularly with my two young children. I had been a smoker since my teenage years, but never had any problems health-wise.

I first went to the doctor in April 2003 because I knew something wasn't right. I didn't know what, but I just knew something wasn't right.

I was getting a pain down my right arm and occasionally in my right armpit and after repeated visits to my GP, I was told to take paracetamol, which I continued to do for some months.

Several months later, I was referred to a physiotherapist as the pain was increasing and becoming more regular. I was asked my occupation and explained that I regularly spoke to customers on the phone, while I typed or wrote down information. I was told it could be possibly neck strain or 'phone-neck' and was given exercises, but they didn't help.

By now, I had been suffering night sweats and going to the toilet during the night. I was also taking paracetamol and ibuprofen four times a day. One evening I was sitting at home and I coughed up blood. I didn't tell anyone about this and looking back I don't understand why I kept this to myself. Was it fear?

One Saturday evening, my wife and I were watching the BBC drama Casualty, set in a hospital accident and emergency department, and one of the characters had the same symptoms as me. This character had coughed up blood, was losing weight and suffering from night sweats. I had been hoping for a diagnosis for the past few months and here I was watching a drama on TV and seeing a character that appeared to have the same symptoms as myself. So I called my doctor on the Monday, but he dismissed my self-diagnosis with *"you don't have cancer"*.

He gave me an appointment to see him and I had a new series of tests yet they still couldn't find what was wrong with me. A few weeks later, I noticed that whenever I had an alcoholic drink, I had an immediate shooting pain in my chest, and I was crippled with pain from just a few sips.

By the November, I started to be worried as I was so fatigued. I went back to see the doctor who referred me to the hospital for an MRI scan; which failed to show anything.

As I was getting myself ready to return to work after the Christmas break, I collapsed on my bed after having a shower. I went to see the doctor again and after taking a blood sample, he discovered my ESR levels were extremely high (while ESR doesn't indicate cancer it may indicate that the body is fighting inflammation or an immune disorder) and he arranged for me to have a CT scan. I was asked to return to the hospital later that day and a consultant would discuss the scan results. I remember he asked if my wife knew how ill I was, which I thought was strange considering I didn't know how ill I was. He suggested they thought it could be one of three things: infection, TB or a tumour. He then ruled out the first two and confirmed I had a tumour: lung cancer. In a way, I was actually relieved to finally find out what was wrong with me.

I've never smoked again since that day.

I drove home and before I could say anything my wife knew by looking into my eyes that what I was about to tell her would change our lives forever. We decided the best approach would be to tell people and not hide it. We were also advised to be honest with our young children but not to scare them.

Due to the proximity of the cancer to my heart, surgery wasn't an option and I quickly started my cancer treatment with weekly chemotherapy followed by radiotherapy sessions.

I was still working and I attended my cancer sessions treating them as if they were customer meetings. I hadn't lost my hair from the chemo so from the outside I didn't look ill, so I just tried to carry on as normal. My focus was getting to the end of my five-month cancer treatment.

At the end of my treatment, my hope had become reality and the cancer had gone. I was classed as NED—No Evidence Detected. The emotions that an NED diagnosis brings are incredibly hard to put into words, and life was about to get back to our new normal.

I was still going for regular scans when it was discovered that new lesions had appeared on my right lung. Unsure what these lesions were, the consultant thought it best for me to have surgery to remove the lung. However, during the surgery they couldn't say for sure if it was cancer and decided not to proceed. Quite soon, lesions began appearing on my other lung and more surgery was needed to take a frozen sample for analysis.

From this sample, they established that cancer had returned. This wasn't lung cancer but Hodgkin's lymphoma and the consultant confirmed it was likely to have been Hodgkin's all along.

It was explained that I would be transferred to a new oncologist, and I would need more chemotherapy. We were advised to go across the road to the Maggie's cancer centre, where my wife picked up a leaflet on Hodgkin's disease and there on the first page she read that one of the symptoms of Hodgkin's disease was an increased sensitivity to the effects of alcohol or pain in the lymph nodes after drinking alcohol. Something I had experienced early in my cancer journey but never thought to mention to my doctor.

My new oncologist painted a bleak picture of the possible outcomes of treatment for this secondary cancer. I was angry because two years later and having been originally misdiagnosed, I was now having to go through it all again.

I was in despair and couldn't see how I could fight this again. I had to hope that the forthcoming treatment would be successful and that the cancer would be gone for good.

I was initially told that they would trial a different type of chemotherapy but after a couple of sessions, they decided it wasn't working and they would need to start a more aggressive chemotherapy, followed by a stem cell transplant.

Over the next few months, I continued my new chemo regime, during which time I was given growth injections to grow my stem cells so they could be harvested and frozen, to be given back to me at a later date.

I was given high dose chemo which flattened my immune system and I had to be kept in isolation in the hospital, as any infection could kill me. During the treatment my body started to break down and I had to be kept on a liquid diet, as the inside of my mouth started to dry out and it became difficult to swallow.

On the third week, my stem cells were re-introduced intravenously. I was also given a drug that they were trialling, which saw me recover and leave hospital much sooner than they had anticipated.

The next few months saw me getting stronger and stronger, mentally and physically, and I was soon able to work on a phased return. This was when it became apparent that I wasn't adjusting to normal life. Things I thought I would know at work, I'd forgotten. I had been so used to being institutionalised and being told what to do, where to be and when that I couldn't cope with the day-to-day routine of the outside world. I had hit the ground with full force with something akin to PTSD.

Thankfully, help was at hand and an appointment was made with a psychiatrist at the hospital. I was told that how I was feeling was completely normal. I attended a handful of sessions where I was allowed to do all the talking about how I was feeling and this really helped.

I had always considered myself to be mentally strong, able to compartmentalise tasks and objectives and beating cancer, twice, I had fallen at the last hurdle.

When I think about what hope means on my cancer journey, I hope that those going through cancer, whether as a patient or family, are offered the support for the physical and mental challenges that you will face.

There are people who can help but the challenge may be finding the right people.

Keith

My Mum Didn't Want to Lose Her Hair

OUR FAMILY BUSINESS STARTED thanks to my beautiful mum, Sue Paxman, who was diagnosed with breast cancer in the 1990s aged thirty-six.

I was only fourteen at the time and my twin brothers were ten; my eldest brother was eighteen.

When mum was diagnosed with cancer, and told she had to go through chemotherapy, the prospect of losing her hair absolutely petrified her. She had the most wonderful head of curly blonde hair, which people would always compliment her on.

Scalp cooling has been around since the 1970s as a way to try and stop a patient's hair falling out due to chemotherapy, but the outcomes were inconsistent and the methods could be torturous.

Scalp cooling works via a number of biological mechanisms that help to limit the impact chemotherapy drugs have on the hair follicle. Lowering the temperature of the scalp causes vasoconstriction, reducing blood flow to about twenty to forty per cent of the normal rate, which significantly reduces the amount of chemotherapy reaching the follicles. To make sure the scalp is reduced to the right temperature, the cap needs to be worn for a period of time before the chemotherapy drug infusion, then during, and for a period of time afterwards, while the drugs are at the most potent in the patient's body.

The method my mum used was very archaic, incredibly uncomfortable and very, very cold.

She tried it at the local hospital in Huddersfield, and unfortunately, it didn't work for her. She woke up one morning to find her pillow covered in hair. This was the first time she had cried since her diagnosis. She had been determined that her children would not see her crying after she was diagnosed, but losing her hair was too much. It was heartbreaking.

As the only girl in the house, she asked me to cut the rest of her hair off. Mum sat in the bathroom and with the orange-handled scissors from the kitchen, I cut off her film star locks and watched them drop to the floor like golden tears.

I felt like I was taking part of my mum away and to this day it is one of the most traumatic things I have experienced. You shouldn't have to do this as a teenager. We both cried and mum made a few jokes and we laughed as the tears and hair tumbled.

Seeing how completely distressed she was by the loss of her hair, my dad Glenn, who was a successful businessman, started to ask questions at the hospital about the success rates of scalp cooling and thought about how it could be improved.

He was told they were trying to cool the scalp, then maintain it at an optimum temperature, which was time consuming and had very limited success.

The process involved using gel caps stored in freezers at the hospital, similar to the sports gel packets athletes use to heal injuries. They were stored for twelve hours before use, removed and the nurses would try to mould them to the patient's head shape, with little success. The gel had to be minus twenty to twenty-five degrees, which is not only difficult to handle, but incredibly uncomfortable for the patients.

As soon as the ice packs were removed from the freezer they would start to warm, making them useful for only twenty to twenty-five minutes. A nurse would then have to leave the patients and go to the freezer to retrieve another pack. This was very time consuming for the nurses, and ineffective for the patient as the scalp temperature would fluctuate. If the packs weren't changed in time, they were less effective.

My dad collected all the information on the current scalp cooling systems and thought, I could come up with something better. He was the managing director of our family business in Huddersfield, which had over eighty years of refrigeration experience. My grandfather Eric had invented the first ice bank beer cooler in the 1950s and the business is still in the drinks cooling industry, supplying innovative cooling solutions to serve beer and other drinks at the right temperature.

My dad thought, we've been cooling liquids for so long, there must be something we can do to improve scalp cooling for mum and other patients. Not long after mum's treatment, he and his brother set about creating the Paxman Scalp Cooling System, which got medical device approval in the UK in 1997.

I often describe our first system looking like something from Doctor Who with rubber Teletubby caps. It wasn't very medical device looking but it ticked the boxes: it was less uncomfortable and less time consuming. That was when the real hard work started, as we had to build clinical data to show that the system was effective, could save staff time, increase the chances of patient hair retention, and was affordable.

At this time my mum's cancer had gone into remission for a while, but not long after she was diagnosed with secondary breast cancer, which had spread to her bones and her liver. She underwent treatment again and used our new scalp cooler. At this time our knowledge of scalp cooling efficacy with different chemo drugs was limited. Mum's drug routine was incredibly harsh and scalp cooling didn't work for her, although she did get some of her hair back quicker after treatment.

Unfortunately, mum passed away at the age of forty-four in October 2000, which is the age I am now.

It was devastating for the family, but her legacy lives on. With my mum's cancer journey as inspiration, we have developed a scalp cooling system used in sixty-five countries. Thousands of patients use these annually during treatment.

This fourth generation scalp cooler is more user-friendly, and due to our efficiencies in refrigeration, it works at higher temperatures to make it more tolerable for patients. Through research, and via testing to ensure a good fit on multiple different head shapes and sizes, we have more comfortable and better fitting caps.

The effectiveness of the scalp cooling is influenced by the type of chemotherapy drug that is administered to the patient. While anthracycline drugs can be challenging, we see the best results with taxane with a seventy to ninety per cent success rate. Success is measured by retaining fifty per cent or more of a patient's hair.

The mental impact of losing your hair is quite traumatic, as I know from seeing how it affected my mum. However, it's not just women who want to stop hair loss during treatment.

Hair loss is in men's top three side effects they want to avoid and treatment affects all your hair. You lose your eyelashes, eyebrows—all your body hair.

Chemotherapy hair loss can be emasculating for men. Simple acts like going to the gym, playing sport and going to work become more difficult when you are conscious of having lost all your hair.

We are a patient-centric business, and everything we do is for the patients. We started this company by trying to give mum some hope. It means so much to us that patients share their stories with us and the positive impact we have had on their lives.

We want scalp cooling to be synonymous with chemotherapy, so that it is offered to everybody. We want it to be accessible for everyone regardless of gender, cancer type, or financial situation and we want to continue to make it as effective as possible.

We are now working closely with Huddersfield University and have opened the world's first scalp cooling research and innovation centre.

The University are cultivating real hair follicles in the lab to understand what happens to them when patients undergo chemotherapy and we're also using 3D printers to develop the ability to produce caps that fit patients exactly.

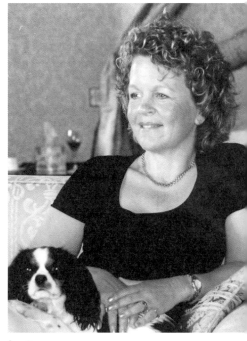

Sue Paxman

Currently, you have a fifty per cent chance of retaining fifty per cent or more of your hair. Through our joint research we are aiming to offer better protection of hair follicles, and our hope is to achieve a minimum of eighty per cent hair retention across all types of chemotherapy treatment that affect hair loss.

Recently, due to an increase in clinical data, we have been able to prove that when you use scalp cooling, your hair will grow back thicker and faster—usually within twelve weeks—even if you have lost a significant amount of hair.

In the UK we work with ninety-eight per cent of public and private hospitals, and also with two leading health home care companies for those people receiving cancer treatment at home.

We know the impact that scalp cooling has on a cancer patient's journey and for those people that hope to not lose their hair, giving hope to more people during their treatment drives us on.

Mum left us twenty- three years ago, but her legacy is giving hope to millions of people.

Claire Paxman

Searching for Hope

I'VE ALWAYS HAD WHAT I SUPPOSE YOU COULD SAY IS A FAIRLY NEGATIVE OUTLOOK on life. I try to have a cup half full but it can quickly flip to being half empty. I try so hard to be happy that I often end up miserable.

I am, honestly, a really nice person—I've just been through quite a lot. And hope isn't exactly something I was used to feeling or looking for.

In August 2012, I was a mum of two lovely boys and, after having been a primary school principal teacher for fifteen years, was on the edge of a five-year career break. Perfect timing to start our own business, an out of school care service that was going to be everything we had always needed but couldn't find. And life was good—actually, really good.

Three months later, in November, I found something—it turned out to be stage 3c melanoma. My breath just stopped.

The plastic surgeons promised it would be dealt with by surgery alone. There was no such thing as adjuvant treatment then—a way to control the spread of melanoma cancer—no treatment to go alongside the surgery. They said chemotherapy doesn't work on melanoma. I had all my surgery—my original primary mole was removed, and the sentinel node biopsy showed cancer had spread to a couple of my lymph nodes, so on to a full lymph node clearance and wide excision of the original site (twenty cm). Then I was sent on my merry way, with three–six monthly check-ups by plastic surgery, and a pat on the head with what I now know are several half-truths to put my mind at rest.

There was no need for hope because I had been told by doctors that I would be fine, so I dutifully believed them. I started breathing again! Indeed, I made sure that it was all put firmly to the back of my mind, almost forgotten.

Life went on, our business was fantastic—I loved it! We were even approached by mums from the neighbouring town to open another service there and we did. In May 2016 we purchased and moved into our own premises—a village hall that felt practically purpose built. I often wonder if we are jinxed. Open a new business and guess what happens?

In July 2016 we went on a camping holiday to Cornwall, as we always do. I felt awful. So tired with a nasty cough and a pain in my side, as if my right lung was catching on something. I brushed it off as being exhausted from working too hard and probably from over-doing it by walking the 26.1 miles of the Moonwalk two weeks earlier. I needed this holiday to rest and get better.

Two weeks of sleep, rest, doing nothing at all, and I actually felt worse. Eventually I almost passed out while visiting Bodmin Jail (and no it wasn't that scary!) so I decided to see a doctor, who told me to go home and go to hospital straight away. I did as I was told, though maybe it was a week later.

Back home I went through A&E at Wishaw General Hospital amazingly quickly because apparently, I had pleurisy and my right lung had collapsed. A week later, the doctors realised I was looking at stage four metastatic malignant melanoma. They told me I really didn't have long left to live. Perhaps three–twelve months if I was lucky, as the cancer had spread inside and outside my lungs, and was completely inoperable. The only thing left for me was to get a permanent chest drain fitted. I would also be referred to the Beatson West of Scotland Cancer Centre but really, it was too late for me.

At that point I just went numb and started feeling absolutely nothing. I'd been told that there was no hope at all.

After two more weeks in Wishaw General, waiting, unable to walk or breathe, my lungs still filled with fluid, I was transferred to the Golden Jubilee in Glasgow which is well known for its excellent heart and lung department.

Then, there it was: a tiny glimmer of hope, when the lung specialist casually mentioned that the Beatson Cancer Centre, where I was headed to next, had a brilliant melanoma oncologist who was completely up-to-date with some positive recent developments in the area. All such information actually passed me by, and the hope was felt with much relief by my husband but I, on the other hand, was still numb to the point of actually feeling quite my normal self on the surface.

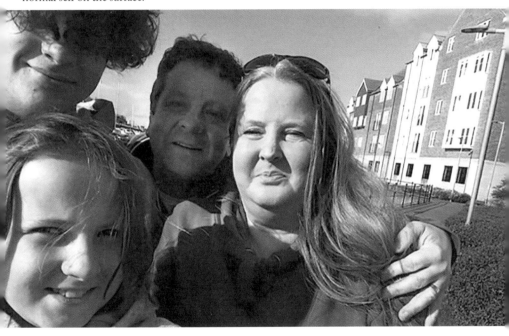

I was constantly being told how amazing I was, how brave, how inspirational etc, because I was the life and soul of the party, doing my usual trick of cracking jokes left, right and centre to cover everything up. What else should I do? Curl up in a ball and cry? I really felt nothing so there was no need for that, was there?

I really wanted to be that positive person, to fight it all the way, blah, blah, blah—but something holds me back. It's actually quite hard to have hope through all this. It's hard to have hope when you are stage four. There is no stage five. What's the point in hope? If the worst comes to the worst I get the easy option—I get to cop out and die.

I have spent all my life having suicidal fantasies and now I am actually going to get to die. The only problem now is that, well, I really don't want to.

On the 23rd of August 2016 (my eldest son's birthday) I started my first treatment—Dabrafenib and Trametinib (Dab/Tram). In a matter of weeks I started to feel a bit better. I could breathe easier.

It was amazing.

Hope! There it was.

But never quite 100%, because this new super-drug was not guaranteed to continue working forever. So we're always going to be living on borrowed time.

My next wee victory?

That my lung had re-inflated and the pleurisy was controlled. Clever lung.

My chest drain could now come out, three months into my melanoma 'journey'. I realised that now I had outlived my initial doctor-given sell-by-date. Then a scan, and the huge news that it looked as if the treatment was actually working!

My tumours were slightly reducing. Now the fight began for real.

The desire to stay positive had crept up on me without me even realising. The longer I stayed okay, the more I started to vaguely think about the future. And there it was again – hope.

The weeks somehow turned into months. Yet still at the back of my mind was the thought that at some point the medication is going to stop working. Living on borrowed time—I was so grateful for the extra time I was being given but please don't take it away from me yet. I was not ready.

The news of another scan. The tumours were continuing to reduce and the treatment was definitely still working.

My emotions were all over the place—one minute hope, the next despair. No wonder I was exhausted!

Plodding along from one day to the next, treading the hamster wheel, taking the meds every day, going to hospital appointments, MacMillan nurse visits, having scans, waiting anxiously for results... then I realise that it has been over 12 months since all this hell had started. I've made it past my final given date.

I'd beaten the clock and was now actually alive within that borrowed time. I felt like jumping for joy, although my physical weaknesses, pain and fatigue would not allow me to do so! So, fight on I must and fight on I will.

The months started to speed by, getting me without much incident to November 2017, although I suffered with Dab/Tram making me very tired. It was decided that I should come off it and try some of the new ground-breaking melanoma treatment: immunotherapy. I was put on a combination of Ipilimumab and Nivolumab. I could only have four attempts with this combination then I would go onto single Nivolumab. So, I had my first infusion and sat back and waited. Five days. That's all it took before I was having excruciating pain in my head and projectile vomiting everywhere. Anti-sickness tablets were a godsend, but the pain didn't go away, rather it built and built and built until I actually felt something blow. Scans showed what looked like brain-lining metastases, and a bleed which used to be my pituitary gland.

It was decided that this combination was not for me! I went back on Dab/Tram as quickly as I could, and everything started to settle back down. I stayed like that through more sets of scans until my brain scans started to show clear again. I have never known relief like it – and there it was again. Hope.

Everything was settled for a while until the end of 2018 when it was decided that the Dab/Tram wasn't really doing much for me anymore and the fatigue and pain was taking over – I could no longer walk without crutches. In January 2019 I very tentatively began a two-year course of Nivolumab immunotherapy (the oncologist obviously had enough faith that I was going to get another good two years then). One infusion each month. That sounded easy, right?

In fact, cancer-wise, it was easy. Routine scans, bloods and MRIs showed that everything either had reduced slightly or at least looked stable every time.

The side-effects, however, I wasn't quite as prepared for! Needing a PICC line because my one remaining vein had closed, developing diabetes, an under-active thyroid, getting Addison's disease, and then the crippling pain and fatigue getting gradually worse after every treatment.

In January 2021 my treatment ended and I went onto the highs and lows of 'watch and wait' which does exactly what it says on the tin.

March 2021 saw what I had been waiting for, for so long. A clear scan. No sign of active disease. I actually had a future, no matter for how long or with what quality of life, I had a future. Hope.

***

Although I am still living with the aftermath of side effects, still with immunotherapy in my system for the next few years, still forever on 'watch and wait', it dawns on me that while I've been sitting here writing this (possibly the most painful essay ever) I have realised how much hope I actually have for the future.

I never had any hope in my life until melanoma cancer came along!

I didn't know how much I needed it until I first felt it. My hope comes in the form of my immediate family, my chosen family, my friends, my house, my business, Melanoma UK, my Melanomamates—my life (in a nutshell).

My life is hope.

There is no need to search for hope. I've found it and it was always there, sitting, watching over me until I was ready for it. And life is there for the taking.

***

"Tired of trying to cram her sparkly star-shaped self into society's beige square holes, she chose to embrace her ridiculous awesomeness and shine like the freaking supernova she was meant to be."

Zoe Houghton

My People are my Hope

MY NAME IS JANE. I am forty-six and have been fit and healthy all my life. I had been having some discomfort in my abdomen (wind, bloating, a feeling of never having emptied myself) from around 2013, which I thought was irritable bowel syndrome. I tolerated it for a long time because sometimes you just do end up coping with low-level irritations.

It got to January of 2018 and I thought I should get it checked out. Around March I saw a very helpful GP who referred me for a colonoscopy and gave me some medication. Nobody, including me, had any idea that it was cancer. The wait for the colonoscopy took seven months. I was told I had a malignant tumour in my bowel and would need prompt surgery and probably chemo. Devastating doesn't even come close to how we felt. I was forty-two, a mum, I had a successful job—my life blew apart and turned grey.

It was initially diagnosed as stage 2 and in November 2018 I had major surgery which I recovered well from. At the end of December it was decided I should have chemo to 'mop up' any rogue cancer cells. The medics seemed quite positive that this would do the trick and then I could manoeuvre out of the cancer cul-de-sac. Hope was there but not in abundance.

I did the chemo (it was horrible) which ended in April 2019. My attitude was, *"Right, I've done my cancer time, let's move on"*. How very naive of me! I returned to work and my actual real, non-cancer, life in May and was very thankful to be able to do this.

Three months later, around the end of July, I had a terrible attack of pain (I thought I was dying or possibly in labour—deeply improbable but I am quite dramatic) in the middle of the night. I was prostrate on the bed, sweating, swearing a little bit and then I was on the toilet. It was awful but I refused my partner to phone an ambulance, as I knew at the back of my mind that it was probably cancer, and I couldn't face it.

I did eventually end up at the hospital having yes, you guessed it, another abdominal op. This time they took out my right ovary which was the size of a small football (thank Christ it wasn't a large one!). What had happened was that an ovarian cyst had swollen up with blood and other 'necrotic' (great word) stuff. Because ovaries aren't properly tethered to your insides, they can twist on the fallopian tube; the pain I had felt was my ovary doing this and then dying as the blood supply cut off—nice!

When they did the biopsy of said small football, they found—lo and behold—loads of bowel cancer cells. I was just absolutely at the end of my mental tether and in total shock (again). Another three months of recovery and rebuilding my life. Clearly the cancer gods felt I had not yet had my fair share of shit.

So, rebuild I did, and returned to normal life around October 2019. I was in multiple shock and not quite myself. The oncology chat was *"scan and monitor"* but as I was *"clear"* of visible cancer, there was no active treatment. Again, I carried on, not really understanding the road I was on. To be fair, no one had given me a bloody map!

And then in early 2020 a scan showed that my remaining left ovary was having the same shenanigans as the other one. It had a cyst that was swelling, so I was booked for an investigative ultrasound.

Lockdown! Ah yes, that thing that happened. The ultrasound was about a week into it and the lady said she was certain I would need surgery again. I wept in the Western's car park on my own. When the fuck was this nightmare going to end? I felt a surge of hopelessness. I knew it was cancer again. The op was scheduled for the end of July–four months of counting the days, uncertain of the future. Lockdown almost didn't really register, it was just another shit thing to endure.

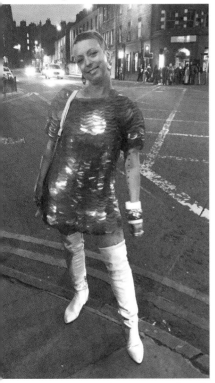

My ovary was weighed, this one was the size of a melon—Galia I believe. Having both ovaries gone put me straight into post menopause: *"do not pass Go, do not collect £200"*. Another gift from the cancer shop. During surgery they found other bits and pieces of suspect tissue and the ovary biopsy showed a small bowel cancer festival occurring. Excellent. By this point, hope was not on my radar, I was just trying to accept the physical reality of recovery again and process the emotional trauma. I still didn't understand the implications of what this turn of events meant, that my cancer had metastasized (tricky word).

And again, I rebuilt my life but by now I was holding onto normality by my fingertips and hope was mostly replaced by dread with lashings of blind panic. I returned to my world around October as things were opening up a bit again. The oncology chat was as before *"watch and wait"* (doesn't fill you with optimism really) which we did until November 2020, when I had my regular CT scan. My oncologist requested an MRI and PET scan about two weeks after the CT. I thought *"Mmmmm, why's that happening?"* but I knew in my gut (what was left of it) and felt barely concealed terror, which I suppressed by getting ready for Christmas—Ho! Ho! Ho!

We had Christmas, which like everyone's was a bit weird and I just knew that something of horror was about to be unleashed on my family once more. Sure enough, we were enlightened at 5pm on Hogmanay—I mean, who schedules these appointments?!

Inoperable. Incurable. Stage four bowel cancer. Seven areas of cancer in my abdomen, one a tumour wrapped around my ureter (a tube for carrying wee). Fear, horror, terror, dread on repeat, relentless. I thought *"Fuck! I'm going to be dead by teatime on the 1st"*. Happy New Year. The presence of hope in our lives was zero.

Everything had locked down again, so I was in a situation where I'd got this diagnosis and was living in our 'dinky' (small) flat, home-schooling our daughter, my partner at the kitchen table doing a stressful social work job and I couldn't cope. I had a breakdown. I visualised my death and funeral non-stop (burial or cremation -the choice is yours). I became obsessed with researching 'cure' stories online. I stopped drinking—that was when I knew shit really had hit the fan! And I was fanatical about food choices/chemicals.

This breakdown lasted about six months and was very hard. But I slowly began to think that there were two options: you live in a perpetual state of doom, turn to the wall and then die—quite a shit option really OR you can live for that day you're in and have hope that you'll be around for the near future—a better option. That is how I live now. I do not let cancer or the treatment get in my way of living. It's not brave, it's just how it is and how I feel.

So, hope. How do I nurture it? Keep it? Where do I get it from? Who do I get it from? My oncologist/giver of hope. Most of the time. He has put me on a combined treatment of chemo and targeted drugs that have shrunk the fuck out of Barbara Twatty (ureter tumour) and her brothers and sisters. That fact alone has restocked my hope supplies but it is a very cautious investment. Barbara's still there hanging about like a last leaver at a party—apparently she'll never go, but she's sitting down and not making a show of herself just now. And that will do.

Medical science is another source of hope for me, as I read quite a bit about new ideas, new trials. But sometimes it can have the opposite effect as many ideas take bloody ages to come to trial or into the wider market and then they're for very specific types of cancer, so I get a bit down about that. But then I start looking at the new frontiers in cancer immunology and cancer vaccines and that makes me feel very hopeful for better treatments, and also a bit superior intellectually—as if! I don't think there will be a universal cure due to the complexity of cancer, but I do have hope that strides will be made in the next decade that will see major changes to cancer treatment and a more multi-layered approach.

Next up is fitness. I don't do sport as that is something other people do, but I have taken up swimming in the North Sea, it is really cold but as far as I know has no great white sharks in it so I'll keep going. The hope comes from the research that cold water swimming boosts your immune system, and boosting that fights cancer, very simplified but that's my take. Also, the coldness obliterates thoughts of any kind, you are just there in the water looking at the sky, fucking freezing.

Then there's the boxing—just training though as I don't want to actually fight anyone, although I'd have a pop at various misogynists and dictators. The other aspect of boxing is the controlled release of anger, of which I have unknown quantities. Very cathartic and cleansing for the soul. And cycling, my great love. My bike is called Vincenzo and we have many wonderful adventures. I have been known to cycle with my chemo pump attached—literally fast tracking that stuff through my body even more to attack the cancer. I'll go up a hill (I don't like hills) but I'll be thinking, *"Fuck you, take that, how do you like it, you horrible piece of me".*

This year I decided to take control of my body by tattooing it. Many things have been done to the good ship Jane, in the name of cancer and its treatments, so it feels quite empowering to mark myself, for myself. They are hopeful marks; they are shapes for each month since I got diagnosed and remind me that I am alive. Some of them commemorate surgeries, people who have died, family birthdays—but they are a constant reminder of how far I've come and to keep going. To never give up. It was recommended that it wasn't ideal to get tattooed while on active treatment, but I did it anyway. I mean, every eleven days I have chemicals put in me that stop my cells dividing so a bit of ink won't even touch the sides. As I write, I am awaiting an oncology meeting which if the chat is good, means I can finish the tattoo marks of September to December 2022. Then I intend to get an anchor on my solar plexus as I consider this symbol to be an international symbol of hope in troubled times—appropriate.

My friend is a great artist and has painted my portrait—starkers—it's artistic though! My chemo pump is plugged into my chest, the point being that I want to show *"here's what living with cancer looks like"*. It's not all lying on the sofa because you're done in from chemo, although that does happen. Projects like this fire me up and keep me enthused about living my life on my terms.

The main thing that keeps my hope going is my people; the love I have felt has been, quite frankly, astonishing. It nourishes my lust for life; it is true that to love and be loved in return is it. I am a very lucky person to have the wealth of humans that I do. They are treasure of the most valuable kind.

Jane Barrow

Hope in a Bag of Apples

"I CAN SEE SHADOWS ON VARIOUS ORGANS."

I heard the doctor say this. A bolt out of the blue, and I was standing in the car park of a local carpet dealer. I had pulled over and quickly climbed out of the car when the doctor asked if I was alone. I wasn't. My thirteen-year-old daughter was with me. I was driving home having just had a scan and I knew then that it must be something serious as I hadn't even got home. Never before had I received a call so quickly from a doctor.

The day before, I had visited an acupuncturist to sort out some lingering back pain. *"Can you look at my stomach too while I'm here?"* I mentioned as an aside. That was when I realised something more serious was wrong. She took one look at the rather lumpy area and found out who my GP was. While I was lying 'relaxing' in her treatment room, she rang my doctor and made an appointment for the following day.

This couldn't be happening to me, to us, to our family. It was the first time I had ever experienced an out-of-body experience and I often think back to this exact moment. I knew that our lives were about to be turned upside down and that this little bump in the road was going to affect us all. My husband and I had four children aged thirteen–sixteen (yes, we have twins!) and we were all going to have to get used to our new normal.

The cancer train is one which, once you're on it, you can't get off... at least not out of choice. I was raced through the main line stations of body scans and joined the platform marked bone marrow biopsy. I toot-tooted through lymph node investigations and one more final scan before being given my diagnosis: Non-Hodgkin's Lymphoma. Blood cancer.

By the time we heard the words, we were relieved. We had been sent down so many wrong tunnels by then and self-diagnosed (usually at 2am) all manner of different cancers. Lymphoma, everyone told us, was a 'good one' to have. Cancer makes you feel so vulnerable, so alone.

The treatment was rough, there's no denying it, but there was also a wonderful sense of camaraderie. I got to know very well my nurses, other patients, and the car park attendant at my local hospital. I would head into hospital at 9am and was usually released by teatime. During all this time I hung on to hope with a vengeance. Hope gave me the power to believe that anything was possible, that we could have a fresh start, a second chance and the opportunity to live life to the max.

During one of my final chemotherapy sessions (I had thirty in total over two and a half years) I came across a wonderful man. It was a really hot autumnal day and an apple farmer wandered into the treatment room in his wellies and shorts. He was huffing and puffing under the weight of bags and bags of apples. He walked up and down the chairs where we were all being treated and, once he had delivered a bag to each patient, he sat down in a chair before being wired up himself. I was sitting opposite him and caught his eye and smiled. He grinned back.

When I stood up to go home, I peeped into my bag. Each patient and every nurse received a bag teeming with delicious, sweet West Country eating apples. It was one of the most thoughtful gifts I was given during all that time. And we all smiled, probably for the first time that day. A smile I remember.

I drove home with the bag of apples on the passenger seat. I know, I know, we aren't supposed to drive after chemo but by then I was quite the professional. My husband had long exhausted 'things to do' in town while I sat for hours and hours on a drip. The gift lifted my spirits and really made me feel great.

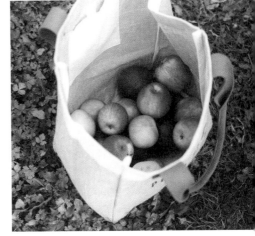

There was something so incredibly uplifting to be given such an unexpected gift without asking for it. I had such a feeling of warmth. Fundamentally the feeling was one of hope. A feeling that said *"I feel your pain, I know what you're going through"*. I felt I wasn't going through this on my own, that so many others cared and I thought to myself, I want others to feel this way.

That was the day 'Treatment Bag' was born. I decided to create a non-profit whose aim was to try and bring this feeling of happiness into the lives of cancer patients. I spent the next year sourcing treats, finding trustees and designing logos.

We now send out hundreds of bags of goodies to men and women having cancer treatment all over the UK. The bags are incredibly popular and we really feel like we are making a difference, bringing some hope into the lives of others.

We now deal daily with many cancer patients, some who receive our bags for free and others who have them given in return for a donation. The act of giving after my own diagnosis has really helped me in my recovery. I come across all sorts of patients from all different walks of life, and I really enjoy hearing their stories of hope. We need each other at such a time, we need to be listened to and we need hope.

So, I'd like to say thank you to that wonderful apple farmer, for giving me the hope and love at a time when I needed it most. I have no idea where he is but if he reads this somewhere near Yeovil in Somerset, I'd like him to know that he has brought happiness and gifts to over a thousand other cancer patients.

A little kindness can definitely go a long way.

Maymie White

A Community of Hope

MY NAME IS **D**IANE, or just Di to my friends, and Crazy Di to my nieces and nephews.
I'm usually the loud one in the middle of the room, the one you hear before you see.

I'm from Liverpool and it might be part of my DNA, but I love talking to people and hearing their story. I'm always curious. Perhaps it was natural that most of my career I've spent working face-to-face with businesses, getting to know them and figuring out how I can help them.

Cancer is something I've always been aware of and in 2013 it rocked our family.

I am the baby of the family, the unexpected child, and growing up I was closer in age to my nieces and nephews than my siblings. My niece and I were very close and every day I remember how she suffered with melanoma.

I watched her fight with every breath until she literally died in front of me. I think back then I really didn't have any hope for anything. She was thirty-eight, beautiful and had her whole life ahead of her and within a blink of an eye, she was gone.

I don't think I will ever get over her death and I wasn't sure what I had to hope for but it's like the film Sliding Doors; you don't get the choice of what lies ahead. Something happens and you go where you are destined to be.

That for me is working for Melanoma UK.

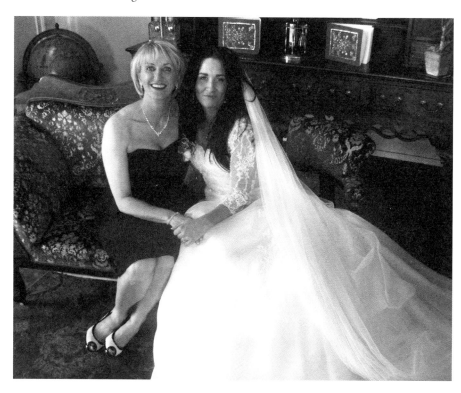

A long time ago I told myself that even on the worst days possible, I have to find just one positive thing to keep me going. The smallest thing keeps me going now, not the big grand things because they are few and far between. I love the small and simple gestures that make me smile. I literally mean that a smile can keep me going and hopeful for what tomorrow will bring.

In my role at Melanoma UK my hope is that I can help patients have a voice, be heard, be supported, and have a safe place to go to during bad and good times. That a patient is heard in every aspect of the work we do. If we don't listen to patients then we cannot do our job and truly support our community.

Historically the patient voice was never heard but this is not the case anymore. We get patients involved in everything we do, we listen, we act and if more than one patient is saying the same thing then we try and do something about it—that's true patient advocacy.

During Covid we started a weekly call with our patient community. One hour every Thursday that's all it has taken to provide additional support and a safe place for patients to openly talk about their highs and lows.

What started out as a four week initiative has now become a regular part of the role we play. No one week is the same. We laugh, we cry, but together we are one big group of hope. The power of this group is amazing. What started out as a patient call has now become a group of amazing friends. Our weekly call is just one way we support the melanoma patient community but seeing our people dealing with major physical and mental issues, but still joining in each week, gives me so much hope for the future.

I know collectively we are so powerful and can give some of our hope to others.

Di Cannon

Hope Comes in Different Ways

AFTER LIVING IN THE USA FOR FOURTEEN YEARS and having several mammograms to check small fibre cysts, there was no alarm or worry when I had a small painful lump on the side of my breast. As a matter of course, I thought, *"I need to get this checked again"*. I had moved back to Edinburgh after a divorce, with my two young sons. My initial thought was that it can only be the same routine as over the pond.

Four weeks later I was called into the doctor's office at the Western General breast unit. Mum sat in the waiting room as I told her, *"Won't be long, then we can go for lunch"*. Within minutes I felt like I had been hit by a train when they hit me with the 'C' word. A breast nurse was also in the room waiting to react to my despair and utter disbelief. Mum was brought in and to this day I can't remember exactly what was said in that room.

My world had collapsed around me. Panic, fear, worry about my two boys had taken over and the tears came and wouldn't stop. We drove home in silence trying to maintain a sense of calm.

Although my thoughts were all over the place, I thought of a mother and grandmother of my son's friends from school who had recently gone through similar. This was the first glimmer of hope that I felt knowing that these two strong women had been through treatment and were living their full life.

Before we got back to Mum and Dad's house my attitude had shifted in the right direction. I think some would call it survival mode. Pure determination to be there for my boys had set in. Hope had kicked in. This wasn't going to stop me. I can do this. Other people had survived this, so why not me?

I never told my boys exactly what I had. They were eight and ten! There was no way I was putting that fear into them. Mum told them I had a sore spot and had to get treatment at the hospital. It was poor timing that a teacher at their school passed away around the same time. I didn't want them to think I was on the same path although the similar hair loss was a big giveaway.

The key to coping was a positive attitude. I looked at each treatment as jumping through the hoops. After each one, it was one less and one step closer to getting my life back. It's strange when you're the one with cancer and it's suddenly akin to driving a car. You're the driver and everyone else is the passenger. They do what they can to help but, in actual fact, you are in control and try to protect them from the outfall.

Some days were dark, leaning over the kitchen sink in the middle of the night, with every joint in your body aching, not being able to swallow due to the metallic taste with silent tears not wanting to wake my sons and letting them see how awful it could get. Despair set in a few times but again grit and determination got me through. Hope was never far away.

It was a year and a month of treatment, with a lumpectomy, seven chemotherapies, forty-five radiotherapies and three further surgeries. I still consider myself lucky as I caught it early and I'm able to give advice to others going through the same thing. To give them hope that they can beat this, and it does get better.

For ten years I had the usual annual check-ups and an appointment with the chemotherapy doctor as I had taken part in a trial with a new drug. Each year the doctor would say *"I wish all my patients were like you"*—that is: no major side effects, clear mammograms, a positive outlook on life to name but a few. It was a comfort knowing that they were still checking and looking out for me. There is a fear that sets in when the treatment is finished and you are out on your own not knowing when it can strike again, if at all.

Finally, after ten years (two years ago), the chemotherapy doctor didn't need to see me again. I was over the moon and still felt good knowing mammograms would take place annually.

Within months, another lump appeared on the same side.

As I sat in that waiting room at the breast unit, I saw the consultant head over to the breast nurse's office. I knew as I sat there what was coming before he even opened his mouth. I was called in with both of them and again hit with the same, *"One of the most aggressive cancers but a different type this time around"*.

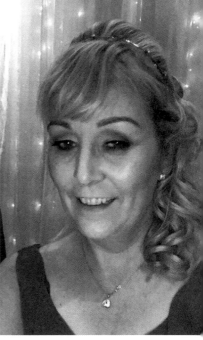

This time a mastectomy was required and four chemotherapies. Apparently, they can't do radiotherapy again on the same side. I was quite shocked at how calm I was. I took it in my stride. I can and will do this again was my first thought. There's no reason why I can't. More hoops to jump through and yes I will be fine at the end of it. I've been here before and I already see the light at the end of the tunnel.

My mastectomy took place in April. I was off for two weeks then back to work full-time. I then had four chemotherapies and I was back working full-time by August. It sounds a bit vain now but I was able to keep most of my hair and I was over the moon. The cold cap was applied during chemotherapy and this freezes your hair follicles to help prevent hair loss. It was excruciating but worth it. That one cup of soup given by the nurses gave me the strength to persevere and keep the cap on.

During this treatment, Covid was rife. My biggest fear was getting Covid during the week that my immune system dropped out. My chemotherapy doctor told me that four patients in the cancer ward had it and all were doing fine. The media were making it to be worse than what was actually happening at the time. This helped to reduce that fear and to continue believing that all will be well.

Hope comes in different ways. Your family and friends keep you sane and help maintain your determination to fight this thing. People you meet during your treatment make you laugh, cry, give advice, give you hope by showing you in small ways that things can get better. Taking one day at a time is key to everything. The breast unit at the Western General in Edinburgh is one of the best in the UK and I am so lucky to have been treated there. The nurses give you hope and the strength to fight every day. They are saints in disguise. I'm thankful for every one of you.

My journey isn't completely over as I have opted now to have the second breast removed. Not sure when, as I still have to get my head around that one. Courage comes to mind. Reconstruction will take place at the same time and I can only hope that it will be the right choice.

Tracey Lipinski

Climbing Out of My Room

I **WAS BORN IN ASCOT IN 2002** and my family then moved to East Lothian, on the coast outside Edinburgh, when I was one year old.

Football has always been my main sport and I went to a high school where we were coached by ex-professionals as part of a programme ran by the Scottish Football Association. From when I woke up to when I went to bed I thought about football. My parents always supported my dream of playing professionally and by 2020 I was playing full-time for Dunfermline Athletic FC in the Scottish Championship. Even though Covid stopped play, I kept myself fit and looked forward to the league restarting.

It was a nice August day and I was down at the beach with my mates when my best mate said the mole on the back of my calf didn't look right. I didn't know what did and didn't look right with moles—I said I'd had it for a while, and it was nothing. He said I should get it checked out. I mentioned this to my mum and dad when I got home. We know our local GP very well—he's a family friend—so my dad took a photo of it and sent it to him.

Covid was still kicking about and we didn't want to bother the local surgery with an appointment for something that was probably nothing.

Our GP got back to my dad quite quickly and said whilst it probably wasn't something to worry about, he'd arrange for it to be removed. I got an appointment to remove it five months later in January 2021.

Life and football carried on and I didn't worry about it, or think too much of it.

January came and I had the mole removed and a biopsy was taken, and they told me they'd be in touch with the results. A few days later when I got that phone call, I was due to go on a second date with Jessica, who's now my girlfriend.

I was quite excited about meeting Jessica, and my mum, after answering the phone, walked into my room with that look on her face. She said she'd just got a phone call asking me to go to the local general hospital that afternoon.

Time stopped. Everything stopped.

I had to contact Jessica and tell her I couldn't make the date and we'd have to re-arrange.

My mum, dad and I drove to the hospital and—due to Covid restrictions—I could only go inside with my mum. We saw a consultant and she said the results of the biopsy was stage two melanoma skin cancer.

As soon as she said those words, my mind and body went into shock. I could see her lips moving and there were noises flowing out of her mouth, but I felt so numb. I still have no idea to this day what she said to me in that room.

Thankfully my mum was able to take some of the information in and ask questions.

Cancer at eighteen.

I didn't cry, there was no emotion in me at that point.

I was staring into the doctor's eyes, probably nodding and making the right noises, but she could have told me I'd won the EuroMillions and I wouldn't have taken it in.

My dad was a big supporter of my career, which was just getting started, and he took the news very badly. He'd been with me all through my football journey and to see it possibly come to an end at age eighteen, hit him quite badly.

We went home and I told my sister and brother that I had stage two cancer and I would need an operation to remove the mole and the area around it. The scariest part was telling them that they didn't know if the cancer had spread to other parts of my body, and we'd have to wait for the results after my operation. Our family is very close, so I knew I had their support, whatever happened.

Our family had already been affected by cancer and loss, as my mum lost her sister before I was born to breast cancer. Both my dad's parents had died from cancer, and he had recently lost his brother in a tragic accident.

The first five days after my diagnosis were the worst.

I sat in my room alone for hours on end, with mum and dad popping in every now and again. There were loads of tears and fears. Will I play football again? Has it spread? Will it kill me? Over those days I convinced myself it was spreading when I slept, and when I woke up it would be in other areas.

I was without any hope.

Those five days were the lowest of my life so far, then something clicked in me—perhaps a survival instinct—and I decided to post on Instagram that I had melanoma cancer and I was going to raise money for charity. Up until then, apart from my immediate family, I had only told my best friend.

I also decided to tell the football club about my diagnosis, and thankfully, they were brilliant. I could have played on until my operation but I knew mentally I wasn't in the right place.

The night before I posted on Instagram, I spoke to my parents and said I want to do something positive. I knew that through my friends and the Scottish football community, I could raise awareness of melanoma cancer, raise money for Melanoma UK, who were already supporting me, and also get into a more positive frame of mind.

It's the best thing I could have done. Suddenly people I didn't know were wishing me well and donating to the charity.

My plan was to climb Ben Lomond, the most southerly Munro in Scotland, with my family. This gave me something to focus on and raised my hopes, that if I did something positive, it might help with my cancer. I also hoped that if I told people what was happening, they could get the facts directly rather than hearing through someone else that I had cancer. I needed to be in control of something to do with my cancer, and I could control the climb and raise money for charity.

I'm always on social media and I'd get a great buzz when I got messages from players at Hearts, who were the team I've always supported. Every positive message helped me to focus on the climb and deal with my cancer.

My initial target was £1,000. I raised over £8,000 with one of my old football clubs donating £2,500, which was amazing.

I did the climb with my mum, dad, sister and our two dogs. It was tough and when I got to the top, looking down on Loch Lomond, I thought I'd feel a great sense of achievement, but it was only when we got back to the car did I feel I'd won this small battle.

After this my thoughts returned to my operation. Before they operated they asked me if I wanted lymph nodes removed from my groin to see if it had spread and I said yes, not knowing if this would affect my career. At that point my hope was that the cancer hadn't spread and I needed to know. That was more important than my football career.

I was quite nervous as I'd never had an operation, or even broken a bone before, and a nurse picked up on this. She started to chat to me, and it turned out her granddaughter was at the same school I had attended, and I knew her. This helped take my mind off the operation.

They successfully removed the cancer from my left calf and took two lymph nodes from my groin, to check if it had spread.

I was told it would take six weeks until they had the results to see if the cancer had spread.

After the operation, the pain in my leg was quite bad and I had to stay in bed for two weeks, which was mentally tough.

Slowly I got out of bed in the third week and had to take my time when I walked. At least two–three times a week I would ask my mum if she thought they'd have the results. I kept badgering her to call the GP, the hospital—anyone that could tell me if I was going to be okay.

Seven weeks later I was walking again and about to leave the house to go and watch my football team play when the home phone went. I was closest to it and I picked it up.

"Hello, is this Cameron?"

"Yes."

"Hi, this is the hospital. The cancer hasn't spread."

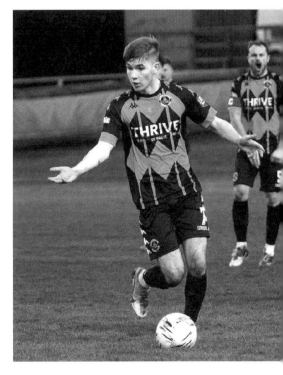

The wave of relief hit me like a hammer. The rush of emotion was immense, and I wanted to tell the world right away. I was calling Jessica, messaging my mates, and shouting to my parents all at the same time.

Joy was spreading very quickly.

Looking back to that time, when I was sat in my room for those five lonely days, I remember saying to my dad that due to the cancer I wouldn't be able to play again. I wouldn't be able to play for the next few seasons, and if I did, I might have to stop playing professionally. I feared the worst and didn't have a lot of hope. No one could tell me it was all going to be okay.

Hearing other people's stories of cancer helped me. One of my former coaches called me when he saw my Instagram post and said he'd had melanoma cancer and assured me I was going to be okay. He shared his story with me.

I wear my heart on my sleeve and if I cried, I didn't care who saw me. There were a lot of tears, but my friends and family were always by my side.

As an ambassador for Melanoma UK, I shared my story and I know it helps other people with cancer. I believe it gives them hope. I get a different satisfaction from this compared to my football.

Right now, I'm happy to see where football takes me. I'm currently playing for Berwick Rangers FC, who despite being from a town in England, they play in the Scottish leagues. As a semi-professional footballer, I'm also working in Edinburgh city centre, living with Jessica, and I have an eye on building my skills and a future career as well as my football.

I hope my cancer doesn't come back and I also hope my story helps other people my age to deal with melanoma and other cancers.

Cameron Graham

Photograph by Ian Runciman

A Degree of Hope

WHEN **L**AURA **WAS** **BORN,** late one long dark night in December 1999, I hoped she would be perfect. She was. I counted my blessings as I counted her tiny toes.

When she started school I hoped that she'd make nice friends, work hard, and enjoy learning lots of new things. She did—and taught me a few things along the way.

When Laura left for university in London, I hoped she'd enjoy her new-found independence, work hard, play hard, and find out what she wanted to do with the rest of her life. Fate, however, had other plans.

When, six weeks later, she called me on an ordinary Monday afternoon to tell me that her trip to the opticians had ended up with an urgent referral to Moorfields Eye Hospital, I hoped it was something and nothing. It wasn't.

Pressure behind the eyes could be a sign of a serious condition but the doctor at Moorfields couldn't see anything particularly amiss and sent her home with a routine referral to a neurologist.

The next day, however, she had the worst headache of her life and was sick all day. Her phone was on silent and I couldn't get in touch with her. As every hour passed, I became more and more anxious until late in the afternoon she rang. Her voice little more than a whisper, *"Can you come?"*

Laura's sister Gracie and I rushed to the station and got the last train from Preston to London, then the tube to Stratford. She wasn't answering her phone again so the security guard from her halls of residence had to use the master key to let us in. We took one look at Laura, curled into a tight ball in the dark of her bedroom and knew this was serious. We asked the security guard where the nearest A&E department was and soon had her bundled into a taxi to Homerton Hospital.

We sat on the hard plastic chairs, fixed to the floor so they couldn't be used at weapons. Laura clutching a cardboard sick bowl and leaning into me as the closest thing to a soft surface available, eyes squeezed tight against the fluorescent lights. I hoped that I wasn't wasting everyone's time and in the same breath I hoped that I was. Crossing my fingers that I was just a neurotic, over-protective mother and this was nothing more than a bog-standard migraine.

Our doctor, Amber, asked Laura to follow her pen-torch with just her eyes, to lift her arms with eyes closed and push against her hand with all the strength she could muster. I held Gracie's hand, hoping Laura was getting all the answers right and that we'd soon be on our way. But Amber requested a CT scan and soon a whistling porter came to push Laura's bed down the dark, empty corridor to the imaging suite, leaving Gracie and I to wait in the silent corridor.

When Amber pulled back the security curtain, she crouched down on her haunches, so her eyes were level with mine as I sat on another plastic chair. I hoped I was misreading the sombre look on her face. *"I'm so sorry but it looks like Laura has a brain tumour, probably two."*

Nobody really expects to hear a diagnosis like that. Brain tumours were plot devices in films and TV shows, a way to explain some dramatic change in personality or kill off a character that had served his or her purpose.

It wasn't something that happened to my eighteen-year-old daughter in her first term at university with her whole life in front of her. All the hopes and dreams I'd had for Laura's future dissolved before my eyes. *"Plot twist,"* said Laura in what was the understatement of the century.

I called a sleep-drunk Mark, Laura's dad, from the hospital's bad news room. The worst phone call imaginable. He had initially thought I was overreacting by rushing down to London but I took no pleasure in proving him wrong. We arranged that he'd drive down to London and together we'd pack up Laura's university room and bring her home. It was so painful. Tears ran down my cheeks as I stripped her bed and boxed up all her belongings she'd lovingly arranged in the tiny room overlooking the Olympic stadium. Her dream was over before it had even begun.

Within a week we had a surgeon and an appointment for a craniotomy. The aggressive growth and Laura's youth suggested that the brain tumours had metastasised from another primary tumour site and so every centimetre of Laura's body had to be examined, as if her body had become a crime scene. It was hard to know what we should hope for: some unknown primary or a glioma in the brain, like choosing between being eaten by a tiger or by a shark.

It felt as if Laura had an unexploded bomb in her head. Only five months ago she'd run her first marathon, two months ago she'd been a political intern working in Chicago and suddenly she was as delicate and fragile as fine china.

On the morning Laura was scheduled for surgery, we couldn't wake her. Her eyes were open but she was unresponsive. Then, as we tried to rouse her, she suffered a huge tonic-clonic seizure rendering her entirely unconscious. Everything was taken out of our hands in a whirlwind of ambulances and emergency rooms with all of us desperately trying to talk Laura back from wherever she'd slipped away to. Fortunately, our brilliant surgeon was still prepared to operate but we'd been warned that, if and when Laura came round, she might not be the same girl.

Those were the longest hours of my life. Hope was all we had, but it was slippery and hard to grasp.

Within twenty-four hours of surgery, Laura was sat up in bed eating mint choc chip ice cream, heavily bandaged and the owner of two spectacular black eyes but she was still Laura. The largest tumour had been successfully de-bulked and fifty neat stitches were already beginning to heal underneath a sterile dressing. She bounced back within days. We were elated, it felt like we had won the battle but in reality this was only an initial skirmish in a long and difficult war.

A week later, we were given a name for the disease: glioblastoma, the most aggressive type of malignant brain tumour and it had spread tentacles across the topography of Laura's brain.

"Like a cancer?" she asked.

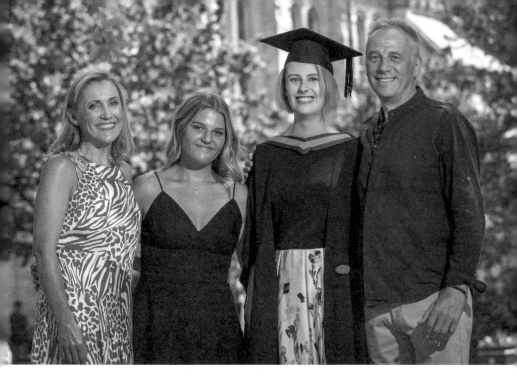

"*Yes, exactly like a cancer,*" the surgeon replied.

She thought about this for a moment. "*Can I go back to university this year or do I need to wait till next year?*"

There was a horribly uncomfortable silence.

"*I'm sorry Laura but you won't be going back to university.*"

The prognosis was twelve months with additional radiotherapy and chemotherapy but just three months without.

I searched online for hope, looking for the right phrase to unlock pages of fantastic new treatments, desperate to read success stories of people living their lives with a gioblastoma diagnosis.

Instead, I learned that treatments for this cancer hadn't changed in decades and although there were innovative new developments in the USA and Germany, there was nothing available to us in the UK. What I didn't realise before this became our life is that brain tumours remain the biggest cancer killer of children and adults under forty and yet receive only two per cent of funding.

Faced with such a grim prognosis and limited treatment options, we manufactured our own hope: talked to experts, raised funds, and tried to heighten the profile of this apparently rare and fatal disease.

We've made the most of the last four years, both by filling our days with adventures from Laura's extensive bucket list and by spending time together as a family, appreciating the simple joy in every day. We are much stronger, more resilient, and braver than ever before.

Our faith in human nature was constantly renewed by kindness. Not just from friends and family but also from complete strangers who learned about Laura's story and offered her days out and experiences that helped us to create truly unforgettable memories.

Laura graduated from the University of Manchester last summer with a 2:1 in Politics, Philosophy and Economics. She graduated right in the middle of the heatwave, and it was a joyous day full of happiness and family pride. She proved her surgeon wrong, just as I'd hoped she would.

It's been no picnic; Laura's had forty fractions of radiotherapy and almost two years of chemotherapy. We have travelled back and forth to Cologne for immunotherapy treatment and in October 2022 Laura had her fourth brain surgery.

Now, when other people look for hope and positive success stories online, they might read about Laura and sometimes they'll even message me. I'm well aware that this is a disease without a cure and at some point our luck will run out but for now we live in hope and try to share that hope whenever we can.

Nicola Nuttall

Song and Dance Man

MY STORY OF HOPE STARTS WITH MY CANCER, but it isn't really about my cancer. I was diagnosed with a GIST (Gastrointestinal Stromal Tumor) in my small bowel in 2019. I was told in 2020 the cancer had spread to my liver and it was incurable.

My prognosis isn't good, but, for now, my treatment is keeping everything stable and the side effects are usually manageable.

I'm a forty-two-year-old father of three young children, living in the north east of England. Before my diagnosis, I spent most of my time working.

When I wasn't working I was, to be frank, drifting through spare time spent with family and friends. I would drink a little, watch boxed sets on TV and, more often than was useful, get myself worked up about politics, football and all manner of other things.

Cancer changed everything in an instant or, I suppose more accurately, my incurable status changed everything in an instant. It was like a switch had been flicked and suddenly I was living an entirely different, much more focused life.

To be clear, cancer isn't my focus. I keep myself as healthy as possible so that I can manage treatment as well as possible—beyond that, my tablets take care of everything until one day, they won't. I'm not going to waste my limited time thinking about it beyond that.

My focus is my family and fundraising (for Children With Cancer UK).

My family need me now more than ever. It sounds like a cliché to talk about making memories and for me it doesn't mean making photo-opportunity memories as much as creating my 'legacy' with my children.

How will they remember me when I'm gone?

How do I want them to remember me?

How can I squeeze decades of parenting into a couple of years!?

I'm not doing anything now that I wouldn't have done before, only now it comes first—everything else is secondary.

My eldest is football mad, so we go to watch as many games as we can squeeze in, and I make sure I don't miss a minute of him playing and training. My two daughters want to make funny dance videos and do crafts, so that's what we do.

When I'm at home I try to be more attentive than I used to be. I cook with love and energy. I sing and dance around the kitchen. That's how I want to be remembered, and that's where my hope comes in.

My wife, Lucy and I, like most families, have been more focussed on the kids than on ourselves for the last many years. It's not easy to roll that back even with my new focus – but I'm trying. We do more things together now and I try to be the best version of me I can be for her. It's not always possible of course, but I try—we try.

My hope isn't for a long life, although obviously I do hope I get as long as possible. My hope isn't for good health—that ship has sailed—although I do hope cancer and treatment stays manageable as long as possible. My real hope isn't for me at all.

I have two hopes and this, in turn is where I find hope.

My first, most personal hope is that I am giving my children—and Lucy—everything they need to live well and happy once I'm gone. I want them to have the tools and the memories they need to meet their own challenges and work through their own battles without me.

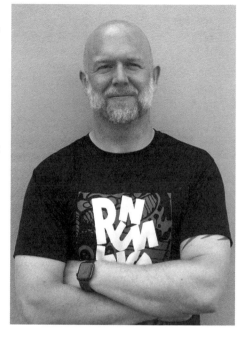

My second hope is for the children and adults who come after me who face cancer. This is where my fundraising activities come in.

My hope is that my small contribution makes a difference and means that in the future, less families have to go through what so many of ours are going through now.

In both cases, I'm working hard to make it work. I'm thankful that I've got a little time to try and when my time is up I'll be able to say I gave it my all.

I won't ever get to see my hope fulfilled, but I guess that's not the point of hope.

Chris Johnson

Snakes and Ladders

LIFE WAS GOING TO CHANGE, and whilst I was apprehensive about leaving Northampton and going to University in Edinburgh at eighteen, I was excited at the prospect of starting a new life. It was the day before we were due to drive up and everything was packed, checked, and ticked off my list.

That morning I got the call that changed my life.

"Hello, are you available to come and see us tomorrow to discuss the mole we removed from your neck?"

My mum had persuaded me to see about a small mole on my neck, which was removed by my GP and now, two weeks later, in which time I had forgotten all about it, they wanted to see me.

"I'm going to Edinburgh to start university tomorrow, so I can't come in."

"Okay, can you come in this afternoon please?"

I agreed to go, and this is the point at which everything changed.

I went in that afternoon and was advised that the mole was stage one melanoma and, whilst they didn't think it was too serious, they wanted to remove a wider area surrounding the mole to check.

So, the day before I was due to start my adult life I was told at the age of eighteen that I had cancer. Whilst the surgery to remove a wider area of my neck would take a few weeks to schedule, my first week at uni was taken up by constant worry about what else they would find and if the cancer had spread. It was a tough decision, but I knew I wasn't enjoying Edinburgh as much as I should have, and I decided to leave the course and take a year off to see what happened.

Over the next year I had the further surgery and scans, and was told the cancer hadn't spread. This was a huge relief and what I had hoped to hear. I then concentrated on finding a university for the next year and enjoying my year out.

In 2007 I started a four year course in Kent and all was going well until in the March of my final year I started to feel incredibly tired all the time, which I initially put down to the pressure of finishing my degree. I had also noticed a lump in my elbow crease.

I was still under the care of my local oncologist back home and when I returned after my course finished, they felt around the area on my elbow and whilst they didn't think it was of any major concern, I was advised I could have it removed if I wanted to.

Having had skin cancer once, I wanted it removed and as it wasn't classed as urgent, I had to wait six months for the procedure.

By the time it was removed in September it had grown a bit bigger and having graduated from university, I had secured my first full time job. I was still living away from home and at the age of twenty-three was fully enjoying life.

Once the lump had been removed, I was told that it was melanoma. I was quickly scheduled for a CT scan. I began to feel as if I was living in a game of snakes and ladders and each time I climbed a ladder, the melanoma Snake was there waiting for me. Whilst I was hoping the scan would come back clear, the thought stayed with me that there was something worse going on.

In late September 2010 I was informed that the results of the scan showed I had lung and brain tumours. Prior to the scan results, I had felt unwell with nose bleeds, headaches and breathlessness. I had Googled my symptoms—which any medical professional will warn you against—just before my scan results and I joked with my boss that I probably had a brain tumour.

When I saw my oncologist, I asked what could be done and the look on his face said it all. There was no sign of hope in his eyes.

"We can try and remove the tumours and we'll do the best we can". At this time there were very few options for melanoma. The current treatments were all designed to try and keep you alive a little bit longer. My cancer had bypassed my lymph nodes, which is usually where melanoma moves to, and this was very rare that it did so.

"We expect you might have one to one and a half years to live." I was twenty-two!

I was put in touch with the palliative care team, which to me seemed like the end of the road, and my family and I began to prepare for my death.

Without initially realising it, I found my next cancer ladder and after the successful removal of the two tumours, I was incredibly fortunate that for the next three years there was no further cancer progression and my scans remained clear. I had beaten the initial estimate, but I knew I wouldn't see thirty.

At this point my hope was that I would be well enough to enjoy life before it was taken from me.

In May 2014, I suffered a lot of severe stomach pains. I was living in London at this time and I walked into my local clinic doubled up in pain and I said I thought I had appendicitis. The nurse asked me some questions. She didn't think it was and when she noticed that it was my birthday that day she apologised for having to send me to the local hospital, which luckily was at the end of my street.

They quickly took me in and tested for various things and noticed that my red blood cell count was really low. They asked me how I got to hospital and I explained I walked from the clinic, which I could tell shocked them. I had five bags of blood transfused over the next two days. I was in hospital for ten days during which they found a blockage in my bowel.

In hospital I couldn't retain any food or nutrients and as I wasn't a registered patient in that health board it was taking time for them to look at my case. I was advised that they would discuss my case at the multi discipline team meeting on the Wednesday. As I had an oncology meeting scheduled at home that same week I asked if I could get discharged to go home and attend my this appointment.

They reluctantly agreed to this and I went home. However, that night due to severe pain, I was admitted to A&E at the hospital my oncologist was based in.

The oncologist came to see me in the morning. He had been in touch with the hospital in London and explained that it might be cancer blocking my bowel. I was scheduled for emergency surgery that morning. The fear was that if it was cancer and it had spread beyond my bowel there was nothing that could be done, and they would just sew me back up and try to make me as comfortable as they could. If they removed the cancer I would probably end up with a stoma for life, which when faced with the other choice was not of any concern to me. If I had a stoma the cancer hadn't spread, and I would live. I was prepared for the stoma, and I had a nurse talk to me before the surgery about living with one. I was quite hopeful at the prospect of doing so.

Another large snake had appeared for me to slip back down.

I had the surgery and when I woke up, I noticed that I didn't have a stoma and there was a very small scar and I immediately thought, *"Oh my god, it's not worked. It is cancer, and it's spread, and they've just sewn me back up"*. My entire world was spinning out of control and one thought was clear: I knew I was going to die very soon and all hope had now gone.

My parents were the first to enter the room. They could see how devastated I looked, and they told me they had spoken to the staff who had told them the surgery went well and they had removed the tumour, that there was no other sign of cancer and they didn't need to remove all of my bowel and give me a stoma.

My emotions flooded the room. After convincing myself that I would die very soon at the age of twenty-four, I now had another ladder of hope.

All through this period I knew that being stage four metastatic melanoma—my official diagnosis—that the cancer could continue to appear and there were no treatments available to stop this or control it once it came back. I had outlived my initial diagnosis and each year I hoped that some form of treatment would be available to keep this monster at bay.

After my surgery I met my oncologist who told me that there was a new drug available for advanced melanoma cancer called Ipilimumab which was an immunotherapy treatment. He wanted to put me on it, but at that time the guidance was that I would have to try another cancer treatment which, if it failed, I could then try.

This was the first time in the UK that there was a drug which targeted melanoma cancer. The ladder in front of me had grown again and I decided to throw the dice and try it.

As we had expected the other treatment didn't work and I was then approved for Ipilimumab. I had two infusions over a four-week period, after which I developed more bowel pains.

I had a scan which showed there was another tumour in my bowel, which hadn't been there at the time of my surgery.

My oncologist said that Ipilimumab would take six months to work based on the early trial data available. We both knew I didn't have this time and it was decided that I try a different drug, which might work quicker, but again was designed to prolong my life a little more.

I was given Vemurafenib, which was a tablet form of cancer treatment for melanoma, which should work quicker than the Ipilimumab. The average time it works is a year and it could work quite quickly.

I chose this little ladder and went to oncology once a month for my prescription and a scan every three months. Amazingly, this treatment worked for nearly two years.

My scans were successful for twenty-one months, then the hospital called me the day after I had another scan. They said they had noticed a blockage in my bowel and asked if I was experiencing any discomfort, which I was. I was asked to go into hospital for surgery that day.

After nearly two years of good health, this continuous game of cancer snakes and ladders had me sliding back down almost to the start again. It's hard to find hope when it keeps being taken from you.

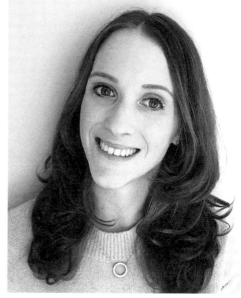

I went back to the hospital that evening and had the surgery, which again didn't leave me with a stoma and yet again they successfully removed the tumour, with no sign of any other cancer.

By this time there was a new immunotherapy drug approved in the UK for melanoma, called Pembrolizumab.

My oncologist said they believed that this treatment has a good chance of extending my life further as there was still no cure for melanoma cancer. The data that was currently available on this new treatment showed a forty per cent success rate, but it was early stages and there was no long-term data.

My life had already been extended a number of times and it felt as if each time I walked down the dark corridor of my cancer treatment, coming ever closer to a dead end, a door would suddenly open for me to present new hope.

I took a forty per cent chance over doing nothing, and was told that I would probably be on this for the rest of my life as, if I came off it, the guidance was that I couldn't get back on the treatment.

Just after I started the treatment, which was an infusion every three weeks, I was approached to appear in a BBC documentary about incurable and terminal cancer. A Time to Live was filmed in October 2016 and featured a number of people that were living with cancer and knew at some point in the very near future, they would die. I decided to take part, as I wanted to leave a legacy for my family. Death was still round the corner for me at this point and my hope was that my family and especially my young brothers would have something to remember me by.

Every three weeks I had my treatment, followed by three monthly scans which continuously showed no new cancer growths. It's hard not to convince yourself that your next scan would show the cancer had returned.

In December 2018, two years after I had started Pembrolizumab, my oncologist told me there's a chance they would take me off the drug, as trial data showed that people on it for two years, who continued to have clear scans, were able to come off it with limited chance of recurrence.

I was again at the bleeding edge of immunotherapy cancer treatment and for once I had just been told due to my continuously clear scans, I might be able to live cancer-free for life. For the past eight years this had never been an option. I was always looking for ways to steal a few extra years and now I could be free?

I went to see my friend who I had known since I was eleven and told her this news. Her jaw dropped to the floor and she screamed, *"What the hell!"* Neither of us could believe it.

Initially I didn't want to stop taking it, as my fear was that I might be the exception to the rule and it was the drug that was stopping the cancer coming back. I was assured that if I did stop and the cancer came back the guidelines had now changed to say that I could go back on it.

I found navigating post-treatment life incredibly difficult. I was told to go and live my life and how could I adjust to this? I was petrified. I owed my life to my oncologist and each time he made the right call.

Writing my story, this is only the second New Year I have thought I'm not going to die this year. I'm now thirty-five and the past seventeen years of my life have been dominated by cancer. I'm not sure if the way I feel about my survival will ever change, as when I hear from friends and work colleagues that they have lost people to cancer I feel guilty. I survived and they didn't.

When I reflect on my journey it blows my mind and looking back, I thought I had hope but perhaps it was just grit, determination and complete faith in my oncologist. I do still question why I'm here and I don't understand why or what the justification is, but I'm just glad I am.

I said this to my friend a while ago, *"It's only the second year I realise I have got my health and I guess the fear of getting ill and dying has subsided, which is amazing and also very scary. I feel very lucky but I'm trying to get my head around and navigate all the shit. I'm so lucky but so many others aren't and life seems to be a toss of a coin."*

She said, *"I totally understand it's a weird thing to not worry, and that I worry about not being worried, that I put myself into harm's way, which is totally normal."*

It's now my job to try and give hope to other people who have convinced themselves that they are going to die. I tell them my snakes and ladders story.

When I started my journey there was no hope to survive, but through a combination of great timing, luck, an amazing oncologist, and research, I had enough time for treatment to catch up with me and for that I will always be incredibly grateful.

I hoped I wouldn't die, even though the odds were incredibly stacked against me, and now I hope I can continue to start living again.

I'm leaving cancer, and I'm not looking over my shoulder.

Jolene Dyke

Thank you

THIS BOOK WOULD NOT HAVE BEEN POSSIBLE without the amazing talent, time, effort and passion of friends, family, professionals, amateurs, and people just lending a hand. Everyone involved in this book willingly gave their time free of charge and didn't want anything in return, apart from the opportunity to help.

I personally know that I wouldn't be the person I am now without the love and support of my wife Sophie, my children Stephen and Katherine, my mum Nancy, my sisters Arlene and Carol, brother-in-law Raymond, and my parents-in-law Frank and Jean, Katrina Armstrong, Helen Lockie and our families. Thank you for helping me navigate my cancer, my treatment through covid lockdowns, and for giving me the hope that tomorrow would be a better day.

For inspiring me to write my story and encouraging others to do the same—in the hope that those who read this will gain something from the stories—I'd like to thank Morag MacLean, Paul Bristow, and Ian Donaghy whose amazing books, The Missing Peace: Creating a Life after Death and A Pocketful of Kindness, gave me not only the start I needed, but an amazing story from Andy Mercer about his brother, Big Boys Don't Cry.

To Derek Watson for presenting the stories and pictures, to Norman Ferguson for the ideas on the layout and his master editing skills, Steve Thorburn for his printing knowledge and Rosamund de la Hey for her publishing guidance. My sister Arlene and my son Stephen for their editing, and my daughter Katherine for the beautiful book cover and illustration. Harriet, James, Olivia, Clara, Rory and Al Russell for proofreading.

Our Melanoma UK family that were always there on a Thursday night for a good laugh, a cry and the odd *"What is Di on about now?"* moments. Thank you, Gill Nuttall and Di Cannon, for making us feel loved. Also, to everyone at Andy's Man Club in Edinburgh for listening.

To Ricky Nicol, Martina Cole, Willie Fairhurst, Steve Langmead and the Commsworld family for their generous donation and helping us to tell these stories, and to Philip Gates, Lara Maudsley, and John Morrison at Morrison Media for sharing them far and wide and to Anne Black for her kind donation.

Thank you also to Kirsty Smith, Mark and Jill Weir, Derek and Julie Watson, Ali and Karen Preston, Matt and Yvonne Barron, Richard and Tanya Elkan, Aonghais and Mairi MacDonald, James and Yvonne Caldwell, Julia Mulloy and Marion Fairbairn, Paul Stewart, Jon Shearer, Marisa Clark-Metcalfe, Ahmed Soliman, Willie Fairhurst, Abid Sadiq, Rory Brannigan, Stephen Milner, Darren Easton, Mark Davidson, Margaret Cudlipp, Mark Curran, Chip Thornalley, Julian Thompson, Grant Porteous, Richard Allenby, Mike Smith, Tony Gribben, Vijay Mistry, Paul Hutchinson, Fraser Anderson, Katie Hughes, Alex Pozzi, Ahmed Soliman, Renato Lilliu, Clive Hailstone, Kenny and Alasdair Godfrey, Alister Richmond, Graeme Watt, Terry Neil, Ian McGowan, Iain Slater, Nick Smith, Richard Shelley, James Tomlinson, Paul Hutchinson, James Morgan, Rob Walton, Rory, Lucy and Clara Doherty, Olivia and Harriet Rafferty. The staff at Borders General Hospital in Melrose, my oncologist

Alan Christie, the staff at the Western General Hospital in Edinburgh and Dr Jim Allison the father of immunotherapy treatment for cancer. Thank you for being there.
To everyone that shared their story with me over a coffee, Zoom or in your own written words—thank you for trusting me.

If you would like to get in touch, please email: **contact@storiesofcancerandhope.co.uk**

Links to cancer charities and other organisations mentioned in the book:

Melanoma UK
melanomauk.org.uk

The Cancer Club
thecancerclub.co.uk

The Treatment Bag
treatmentbag.co.uk

Maggie's
maggies.org

Macmillan Cancer Support
macmillan.org.uk

Andy's Man Club
andysmanclub.co.uk

The Mulberry Centre
themulberrycentre.co.uk

Teenage Cancer Trust
teenagecancertrust.org

Children with Cancer UK
childrenwithcancer.org.uk

Move Against Cancer
movecharity.org

Ian Donaghy
bigian.co.uk

Cold Cap
coldcap.com/stories